THE SAGA OF THE
TIJUANA BARBELL CLUB

THE SAGA OF THE
TIJUANA BARBELL CLUB

JOSH BRYANT AND ADAM BENSHEA

THE SAGA OF THE TIJUANA BARBELL CLUB

JoshStrength, LLC and Adam benShea

Copyright © 2017

WARNING! - Before starting any training program, please consult your doctor or other health care professional. You are agreeing to take full responsibility for any potential risk associated with anything put into practice from this book.

For further explanations and demonstrations regarding the workout programs in this book, please refer to the video collection on our YouTube channel: https://www.youtube.com/user/jailhousestrong

Dedicated to Charles R. Poliquin, who embodies physical culture, drinks deeply from life, and teaches by example.

TABLE OF CONTENTS

PREFACE

Every memorable story exists at the intersection of truth and imagination. The Saga of the Tijuana Barbell Club is no different. As time has woven its colorful thread into our shared memories, it is increasingly difficult to separate fact from fiction. Rather than attempting to nitpick our way through our remembered past, we decided to accept the mosaic created by the narrative and to use the story as a means to improve our training, our lives, and our relationship with those around us.

We suggest that you do the same. Use this story as much as it serves you.

THE ORIGINAL MEMBERS OF THE TIJUANA BARBELL CLUB
Chato: The narrator of the Saga of the Tijuana Barbell Club. He is named for the Chiricahua Apache chief and his face bears the genetic imprint of a native heritage. Although younger than the legendary lifters at the Tijuana Barbell Club, he was old enough to internalize the strength lessons, put them into practice, and remember them.

Charuto: With a naturally tall and slender build (the reason that he was called 'Cigar'), through diligent training he turned around his composition and the direction of his life. He became a legendary bouncer and strongman.

Oso: A large (and very hairy) man who said little but trained hard and often. He was the primary spotter for Charuto. At times, he was mistaken for the Mexican Bigfoot.

Kirk Peters: An all-American jock who was spending some time in Old Mexico before continuing with the seminary. He is called to serve his flock, but he feels that he must first have his experience in Tijuana. Central to that experience is the development of physical strength and working alongside Charuto at the bar. During his tenure at the bar, he becomes the best bouncer in Tijuana.

INTRODUCTION

The age of adolescence is a formative time. Your teenage years are filled with experiences that will entertain you, haunt you, inspire you, and continue to influence your personal development. During this period, you are making the transition from childhood to adulthood. In the midst of this transformative process, you are searching continuously for a story, or myth, that will infuse your developing life with meaning, purpose, and direction.

You never know where you will find a narrative with the force sufficient to influence the path of your life. Maybe it was the stories from your merchant marine, power drinking uncle that left an impression. Many find importance in the action movies of the 1980s or the gangster rap lyrics of the early 1990s. Others may look to the biographies in Plutarch's *Lives* or the Horatio Alger novels of the 19th century. Whether you are considering the tale of Dalton in *Roadhouse* or the conquests of the Macedonian Alexander the Great, what's important is that you found narratives to use as navigational points during the trajectory of your life.

For us, a central element of our teenage years was the local gym where we trained. If you were hunting for stories, this was a target-rich environment. In one corner of the gym, you would find a retired CIA case officer who was living out of his van, warning people about the looming Y2K crash, and occasionally challenging other lifters to a gun duel in the parking lot. In another corner, bulked up bouncers from the local strip club thumbed through pages of a muscle magazine while discussing the benefits and detriments of different supplements. Over near the dumbbells, a middle-aged, ex-high school gridiron star, who still lived at home, complained about the Persian mechanic who stole his girlfriend while simultaneously dishing out relationship advice. Under the pull up bar, a gay bodybuilder, who made millions designing water features for outdoor gardens, chatted up an aspiring movie producer about the shifting social dynamics of the local film festival.

There was quite the cast of characters all sharing a lively exchange of eclectic stories. And unsurprisingly, the din of this chatter would often rival the clank of the pig iron. Amidst this noise, there was an older lifter who remained off to the side.

He was removed but not apart from the happenings at our gym.

By his weather-beaten face, you could put him at well over 60 years old, and maybe as old as 80. From the breadth of his shoulders and a torso rippled by hours of hard training, you would assume that he was much younger. While his face bore the imprint of a rugged life, there remained an aquiline nobility to his features. The young and inexperienced gym-goers paid him no mind. The older and broader lifters treated him with a quiet reverence. Sometimes the old-timers would nod or exchange a few words with the man, but few stayed in his company for long. You got the impression that he possessed an intensity that made some uneasy and many uncomfortable.

For us, the gym was a place to lift as a means to improve our performance for the next football season or wrestling year. Our dedication to training meant that we would often train late into the night, when most others would have trickled out to their evenings of family responsibilities or night club gatherings. On one particular night, the gym was nearly empty. Without the seemingly endless chatter of an overflowing training hall, a cathedral-like hush floated lightly above the weight room.

Our focus on finishing a set of close grip bench presses clouded our peripheral awareness and we were unaware that the mysterious old stranger locked us in his gaze. He must have moved with a cat-like quiet because before we knew it, he crossed the length of the gym and stood alongside us. Before he spoke, you could feel his presence. He had a significant amount of presence.

His face, deeply creased by scars and time, resembled a worn topographical map and you traversed those deep slopes to reach eyes that were curiously both gentle and hardened. In a way, he was a study in opposites. A wizened face with a youthful explosiveness in his movements. A man who captured attention with ease, but preferred an inconspicuous place in the corner of a room.

"You kids are here pretty late. Don't you have girls to chase or video games to play?"

"We don't play video games," we replied in near unison.

"What about girls? You kids make time for girls, right?"

We chuckled and nodded in confirmation.

"Good. You know, I have been watching your training. You kids train with an intensity and regularity that reminds me of one of the greatest periods in physical culture." As he said this, his eyes wandered off to the horizon. "I am not talking about Venice in the 70s. Well before that, there were some real training down in Tijuana."

"Tijuana?? The place known for jell-o shots and strip shows?"

With a slight smile and an almost imperceptible nod, he replied, "Well, that's part of the city's history." Some of the humor left his face and his leathered skin tightened with his sincerity. "Another part of the city's history are the old time strongmen of the Tijuana Barbell Club. I am going to tell you kids a story. I will share the experiences of these men because whenever their story is told, it keeps them alive for another generation. I am also telling you this story because you kids seem like worthy trustees of their training philosophy."

With this encounter, we were drawn into the saga of the Tijuana Barbell Club and now we are sharing this story with you.

CHAPTER ONE
THE ORIGINS OF CHARUTO
AND CLUSTER SETS

A couple of days after this initial meeting, we headed over to the gym to complete our workout. But as we pulled up, we saw a billowing blue tent covering the entire gym. It looked more like a Ringling Brothers Circus than a training facility. Taped to the section of the tent, where the door would be, we found a note:

> *Due to a slight termite problem. This facility is being fumigated. As a consequence, the business will be closed for the remainder of the week. We apologize for any inconvenience.*

At a loss for words, we looked at each other and wondered what we would do. How would we train? Maybe, the commercial gym downtown would offer us some sort of week-long membership. Failing that, we could head over to the high school and see if we could scrap together a workout on their equipment.

While mulling over our options, we felt a presence behind us and turned to see the same old lifter from the other day. We did not see or hear any car drive into the lot. Did he walk here?

"I thought that you guys would be here. I can't imagine that you'd let some pest control get in the way of training. You can't let too much get in the way of your training."

"We didn't know about this and were just talking about where we could train."

"Well, the owner, Greg, left some old equipment on the outside of the gym, along the side. He probably thought that nobody would want to use it. He forgets that old diehards like me won't skip a workout and know how to make the most of minimal equipment. I'll show you."

As we followed, we realized that we did not know his name and asked as much.

"They call me Chato."

"Like the old movie Charles Bronson?" We asked.

He gave a slight chuckle. "Well before that movie, there was a famous Chiricahua Apache chief by the same name. Legend has it that I have some Apache blood in me and so Charuto gave me the nickname. Charuto had a nickname for everyone in the Tijuana Barbell Club down in Old Mexico, everyone except Kirk Peters. He did not need anything beyond what God gave him."

"Who is Charuto?"

"Charuto was the founder of the Tijuana Barbell Club and at one point he was known from Tijuana to San Felipe as the best bouncer in Northern Baja. Just about everything that I know about lifting, I learned from him."

"What about Kirk Peters? Who is that?"

"Well, that's another story entirely."

While talking, we arrived upon some dusty old equipment arranged along the side of the gym. To say the set up was spartan would be an understatement.

There was a pull up and dip tower, an array of dumbbells, and an old barbell with some rusty plates.

Surveying the iron, Chato's eyes seemed to be looking back to another time, another place.

"You know, Charuto started lifting with a set up not too different form this. He was a street kid in Tijuana. He came from a long line of *campesinos*, or peasant farmers, down in the rugged mountains of Sinaloa. When the crops started to dry up, his family moved to Tijuana.

"He didn't get much to eat as a kid, so he was real skinny. Long and lean. Like a cigar. That's how he got his nickname, *Charuto*.

"But, the thing about Charuto was that he was going to be defined not by where he came from, but where he was going. One night while loitering on the streets of Tijuana, he caught his first glimpse of those neon lights of the night life. Charuto, this skinny street urchin, saw a broad shouldered, barrel chested bouncer work the door. For Charuto, this man was the picture of everything he was not. The bouncer was strong, confident, and respected by all those around him. He look regal.

"At that moment, Charuto saw what he wanted to become: a man of strength and confidence. He had no money, but he knew how to hustle. Doing everything from selling cheap gum to picking up tacos for the neighborhood *jefe*, or boss, he scrounged together enough *pesos* to buy some old weights and with an old blue tarp as a makeshift roof, the original Tijuana Barbell Club was established.

"Without much equipment, he knew that he had to make the most of what he had. So he came up with this cluster set workout, which became the starting point for his physical transformation from an unknown street kid to a legendary bouncer and strongman. Eventually he would work the door at some of Tijuana's bars, like the old Nelson Bar and El Dandy del Sur between Revolucion and Madero avenues. And once, he was contracted by the famous Kentucky Club in Juarez to guard Frank Sinatra.

"Perhaps the greatest lesson I learned from Charuto is this: *Do not let your genetic makeup define your destiny.*"

We were completely mesmerized by this story and eagerly asked about the details of the cluster workout.

Cluster sets are those in which the main sets are broken into several parts. For example, instead of doing a set of nine reps you do a set of 3+3+3, which allows for a very short rest period within the set. That intraset rest period allows you to lift more total weight for more sets. This offers a great anabolic stimulus. If you are looking for muscle growth, the rest period can be very short, but no more than about 20 seconds.

In this workout, you pick a weight that you are capable of handling for 10-15 reps. Lift the weight for five reps, rest 15 seconds, and repeat the sequence; do this for five minutes straight. If you can no longer do five reps, drop it to four reps; if you can no longer do four reps, continue with three reps. If three reps becomes unmanageable, lengthen the rest interval to 20 seconds; if this becomes too much, stop the set and move on to the next exercise. On the last set, if you have gas left in the tank, take that set for as many reps as possible.

All that you need for an arm cluster workout is a pull up and dip tower, some dumbbells, and a barbell. This workout can be performed once a week as part of a traditional bodybuilding split or twice a week if you are specifically working to bringing up lagging arms.

No rest is required between exercises, since you are alternating between biceps and triceps. Make sure to perform a warm-up set or two before starting the cluster sets.

One of the benefits of cluster sets is that they allow you to accomplish more volume in less time.

Exercise	Workout
Dips	Cluster
Chin-ups	Cluster
Incline Barbell Triceps Extension	Cluster

Barbell Curls Lying against an Incline	Cluster
Tate Press	Cluster
Hammer Curls	Cluster

This was the first cluster workout that we learned from Chato. Over time, we learned about a number of different types of cluster workouts. One of the important features of this training is that there should be minimal rest between exercises. The only rest should be during the time it takes to transition from one movement and set up the next one.

With the workouts adapted from Chato's teachings (described below), do not perform the same exercises more than four weeks in a row. You can alternate movements by using the provided substitutions.

CLUSTER SET ARM WORKOUT

Exercise	Workout
*Dips	Cluster
**Chin-up	Cluster
***Overhead Rope Triceps Extension	Cluster
****Barbell Curls Lying against an Incline	Cluster
*****Dumbbell Floor Triceps Extension	Cluster
******Hammer Curls	Cluster

Exercise Notes

*Add additional weight if needed. Only do dips if you have equipment that allows for an easy/efficient set up. Possible substitutions for dips: seated machine dips, close grip push-ups, Smith machine close grip bench press, close grip bench press, or Kaz press.

**Add additional weight if needed. Only do chin-ups if you have equipment that allows for an easy/efficient set up. Possible substitutions for chin-ups: reverse grip lat pulldowns, barbell curls, standing/seated cable curls, or Scott curls barbell or dumbbell.

***A triceps v-handle or cambered attachment is fine, but a rope is preferred if you have access to one. Possible substitutions for overhead rope triceps extensions: French press, seated dumbbell overhead triceps extension, triceps rope pushdown, or bodyweight triceps extensions.

****Make sure the incline is set so the barbell is easy to grab in the bottom position and check for any obstructions on the incline that would not allow for performing this movement with a full range of motion. Possible substitutions for barbell curls lying against an incline: machine curls, barbell curls, incline dumbbell curls, Scott curls barbell or dumbbell, or standing/seated cable curls.

***** Stop each rep for approximately a quarter of a second, just long enough to break momentum. Possible substitutions for dumbbell floor triceps extension: seated machine dips, close grip push-ups, smith machine close grip bench press, close grip bench press, or Kaz press.

******Each rep is performed in a "dual action," i.e., lifting both arms at once. Possible substitutions for hammer curls: reverse curls, rope hammer curls on cable stack, towel kettlebell curls, Zottman curls, or incline hammer curls.

CLUSTER SET SHOULDER WORKOUT

Exercise	Workout
*Machine Military Press	Cluster
**Lateral Raise	Cluster
***Rear Delt Fly	Cluster
****Face Pulls	Cluster
*****Plate Raise	Cluster

Exercise Notes

*Our preferred machine for this exercise is hammer strength, but any machine that allows for minimal time setting up will work. A barbell is okay only if it is set up on safety pins in the power rack, to avoid wasting timing. Unless you have power hooks, do not use dumbbells because they can be cumbersome. Possible substitutions for machine military press: any seated or standing machine military press, barbell presses that fit the described criteria, or landmine presses.

**Use any machine or dumbbells that allow for easy set up. A possible substitution for lateral raises is any machine or dumbbell that makes the set up easy and allow contraction for both sides simultaneously.

***Any machine that allows you to perform a reverse fly for the rear delt will work as long as set up is efficient. Possible substitutions for rear delt fly: bent over dumbbell reverse fly, face down incline dumbbell reverse fly, incline face down wide grip front raises, or band pull aparts.

****To perform a face pull, attach a triceps rope or push down strap (a band may also be used) to the high attachment on a lat machine. Step back and place one foot on the seat for support. Next, pull the rope toward your face with your elbow out. As you pull the rope back, squeeze your shoulder blades together. Possible substitutions for face pulls: bent over dumbbell reverse fly, face down incline dumbbell reverse fly, incline face down wide grip front raises, and band pull aparts.

*****Perform plate raises by completing the following steps:

1. While standing straight, hold a barbell plate in both hands at the 3 and 9 o'clock

positions. Your palms should be facing each other and your arms should remain about 15 degrees short of lockout throughout the duration of the exercise. At the beginning of the movement, the plate should be down near your waist in front of you.

2. Raise the plate up from your waist to eye level. Your torso should remain stationary throughout the movement.

3. At a controlled speed, lower the plate back down to the starting position.

4. Repeat for the recommended amount of repetitions.

Possible substitutions for plate raises: dumbbell front raises standing or seated, cable front raises, or lying front raises.

CLUSTER SET LEG WORKOUT

Exercise	Workout
*Squats	5, 3, 1
**Romanian Deadlifts	6, 6, 8
***Leg Press	Cluster
****Leg Curls Lying	Cluster
*****Leg Extensions	Cluster

Exercise Notes

*Perform full squats as heavy as possible; progressively increase the weight used each set. Take a full recovery between sets. Possible substitutions for squats: safety squats, front squats, Zercher squats, box squats, or squats against band or chain resistance.

** Perform deadlifts as heavy as possible; progressively increase the weight used during each set. Take a full recovery between sets. Possible substitutions for Romanian deadlifts: one leg Romanian deadlifts barbell or dumbbells, split stance Romanian dumbbells, good mornings, deadlifts, or glute ham raises.

***Use a full range of motion. Possible substitutions for leg press: hack squats, sissy squats, any leg press variation or alternate leg press machine, or pit shark belt squats.

****Advanced athletes can perform these cluster sets with three reps, with an eight repetition max. This is because the hamstrings are predominantly fast twitch and react better to lower reps. Possible substitutions for leg curls lying: glute ham raises, leg curls seated, cable Romanian deadlifts, slider leg curls, TRX leg curls, or stability ball leg curls.

*****Avoid any cheat reps on this exercise! Possible substitutions for leg extensions: hack squats, sissy squats, any leg press variation or alternate leg press machine, pit shark belt squats, or bodyweight squats.

CLUSTER SET BACK WORKOUT

Exercise	Workout
*Deadlifts	5, 3, 1
**Tbar Prison Rows	Cluster
***Wide Grip Pull-ups	Cluster
****Seated Rows	Cluster
*****Narrow Grip Neutral Grip Pull-ups	Cluster

Exercise Notes

*Perform deadlifts as heavy as possible; progressively increase the weight used for each set. Take a full recovery between sets. Possible substitutions for deadlifts: rack pulls, deficit deadlifts, trap bar deadlifts, or farmer's walk with three sets for 20 yards and as much weight as possible

**Perform T-bar prison row by completing the following steps:

1. Place the end of an empty barbell into the corner of a room.
2. Rest a heavy dumbbell or some weight plates on it to hold it down.
3. Load the opposite end of the bar with plates and straddle it, using a narrow neutral grip handle.
4. Bend over at the hips until your torso is about a 45-degree angle to the floor with

arms extended and then pull toward your chest.

Possible substitutions for T-bar prison rows: seated rows, plate loaded chest supported rows, seal rows barbell or dumbbell, or Yates rows.

***Add extra weight when applicable. If needed, band assistance can be used. Possible substitutions for wide grip pull-ups: wide grip lat pulldowns, cable lat pulldowns, nautilus pull overs, machine assisted pull-ups, or neutral grip pull ups.

****Use a neutral grip handle. Possible substitutions for seated rows: standing cable rows, plate loaded chest supported rows, seal rows barbell or dumbbell, or Yates rows.

*****Add extra weight when applicable. If needed, band assistance can be used. Possible substitutions for neutral grip pull ups: neutral grip lat pulldowns, cable lat pulldowns, band lat pulldowns, machine assisted pull ups, or wide grip pull-ups

CLUSTER SET CHEST WORKOUT

Exercise	Workout
*Bench Press	5, 3, 10
**Push-ups	Cluster
***Machine Incline Press	Cluster

| ****Seated Cable Fly | Cluster |
| ***** Incline Cable Fly | Cluster |

Exercise Notes

*Go as heavy as possible each set. Possible substitutions for bench press: incline press barbell or dumbbell, decline press barbell or dumbbell, dumbbell bench press, or weighted dips.

**Additional resistance can be added via a weighted vest or resistance bands. Possible substitutions for push-ups: dips, any incline, decline or flat press machine variation, push-ups on the knees, feet elevated push-ups, or push-ups against the wall.

***Hammer strength is our preferred machine. Possible substitutions for machine incline press: any variation on a machine, Smith machine reverse grip bench press, dumbbell reverse grip bench press, or feet elevated push-ups.

****Hold each rep a half-second at the contracted position. Possible substitutions for seated cable fly: pec deck machine, dumbbell fly, or standing band fly.

*****Hold each rep a half-second at the contracted position. Possible substitutions for incline cable fly: feet elevated push-ups, incline dumbbell fly, or incline band fly.

Chapter Two
Body Types and
Individualism

Chato was not the only friend we made at the gym. In those days, we spent a lot of time talking with an eclectic array of characters who gathered around the iron. On one particular evening, a doorman from the local strip club wanted to share a workout from a lifting magazine. He passed along the article for us to read.

While we hovered over the magazine, Chato walked to us and asked what we were reading. We showed him and as he started to read the article, his lips moved slowly and silently pronouncing each word. After a few moments, his face showed a growing sadness.

Up until this moment, Chato had not revealed much emotion. So, at a loss for words, we remained quiet and anxiously waited for what came next.

His powerful profile stared off to the horizon. After some time his face turned and his intense stare met our eyes.

"You know one of the saddest things that I have seen?"

We were too young to know an answer, but old enough to know not to give a silly reply.

He took our silence as an invitation to continue and did so: "It is a sorry sight whenever you see someone sacrifice their individuality. *The one thing worth anything in this life is YOUR individual spirit.* In my view, anything that looks to stifle your individual spirit is inherently wrong.

"While it may have some good ideas, this article is packaged for mass consumption like those emaciated mechanically raised chickens sold in chain franchises.

"You boys are worthy of better quality. You must train in the same manner that you live your life. The path you follow should be as unique as your particular nature."

This was some deep stuff and he could tell from the looks on our faces that we were processing what he said, but we needed to hear more.

"I am not saying that you live a life of reckless abandon for rules or morals. I am saying that you must find a plan, then walk a path that works for you. Do not just pull from the assembly line, because you guys are better than that."

Still astonished by the intensity of the words and his stare, we muttered a somewhat incomprehensible question asking him how he learned this way of thinking.

"Like many of the most important lessons in my life, I learned this at the Tijuana Barbell Club.

"You see, the Barbell Club started small, but Charuto continued to save his money and bought some more equipment. He found an abandoned structure in the borough of Playas de Tijuana, not far from the beach, and moved his weights into that place. Some nights, when the winds were right, you could hear the breaking surf and smell the salt water.

"With a good location and growing pile of iron, Charuto found some partners to train with. First come Oso, who got his name because he was large and hairy, like a bear. While Charuto was naturally thin, Oso was naturally chubby. But both trained hard and developed their bodies into massive mountains of muscle. And they put that muscle to work at the beer halls of Tijuana, Rosarito, and Ensenada.

"With time, Oso and Charuto developed a reputation in the bars around the northern Baja of Old Mexico. Then, one day when the sky was a celestial blue and streaks of sunlight shot down from the heavens, there came a *gringo* from across the border. Kirk Peters was his name. Oso and Charuto, they came from the streets and any education that they hard was learned there. Kirk Peters, he was educated in a more traditional manner. We learned later that he was a theology student, who one day walked out of the seminary. He said he needed some time to learn things that are not found inside of a library and he came to Old Mexico because he needed some time to breathe.

"I still remember the first day his well-proportioned frame filled the doorway of the Barbell Club. You could see the ocean far off in the distance behind him and he had this broad smile across his face, like he just knew that he found what he was looking for. He started training alongside Charuto and Oso. Now they all trained together, but they trained differently. Where Charuto and Oso were overcoming their genetics, Kirk Peters was gifted with a beautiful natural physique."

"So how did each of them train differently?" we asked.

"They each chose a training model that worked with their particular body type."

When developing or choosing a workout program, one of the first things to recognize is your particular body type.

The late psychologist, William Sheldon (1898-1977), life's work consisted of observing human bodies. These observations led Sheldon to classify three distinct body types, known as somatotypes. The three somatotypes are the ectomorph, endomorph, and mesomorph. While most people are a combination of two somatotypes, it is important to first identify characteristics of each type and then figure out the training method that best serves each type.

ECTOMORPH TRAITS

Charuto's build would be classified as the ectomorph type. The ectomorph is the proverbial "hard gainer" (but Charuto did not let this stand in the way of his training goals). Some general traits are: a flat chest, small shoulders, thin, small joints, droopy shoulders, long fingers, long toes, and long skinny neck. On the upside from a physique standpoint, ectomorphs are relatively lean.

ECTOMORPH CHALLENGES
Ectomorphs have an extremely efficient metabolism. They are at a disadvantage for bodybuilding training because their fast metabolism kills potential muscle gains.

Conventional wisdom holds that if you are having trouble gaining muscle, increase your caloric intake by 500 calories per day.

ECTOMORPH TRAINING TIPS
Being an ectomorph is not a sentence to mediocre muscular development purgatory! Follow these training tools to breakout of what some consider a genetic prison and be thankful that you are naturally lean.

- Train with 10+ sets per body part.
- Can train muscle groups more frequently than endo- or mesomorphs (generally need about 2/3 the recovery time of a mesomorph).
- Train with 15+ reps per sets, often.
- Avoid aerobic training.
- Missing a meal is much worse than having a bad meal.

- Many ectomorphs suffer from an anxiety and this halts weight gain. Consider supplementation with Phosphatidylcholine.

ECTOMORPH TRAINING FREQUENCY GUIDELINE

Ectomorphs are the hardest gainers, so they can train more often and with more volume than mesomorphs and even easier gaining endomorphs. The number of days of rest recommended for each body part before training it again is as follows:

	Days of Rest "Light Day"	Days of Rest "Medium Day"	Days of Rest "Heavy Day"
Large Muscle Groups: • Upper Legs • Lower Back	3	4	5
Medium Size Muscle Groups: • Chest • Upper Back • Biceps • Triceps • Shoulders	2	3	4
Smaller Muscle Groups: • Midsection • Calves • Forearms	1	2	3

ENDOMORPH TRAITS

With his ursine, or bear-like, build, Oso was a classic endomorph. Endomorphs can be classified by soft and round bodies. Before weight training, their muscles are very underdeveloped. Endomorphs are identified by a very robust girth. Generally, the arms and legs of an endomorph are short in length, further exacerbating the look of a squat, short individual.

ENDOMORPH CHALLENGES

The good news is endomorphs can pack on muscle fairly easily. The bad news is this body type is prone to excessive accumulation of body fat, especially in the form of a large "spare tire" in the midsection.

Low carb diets will produce vastly superior results for the endomorph. Along with a fairly high dietary fat consumption, protein consumption should be over one gram per day. A great place to start nutritionally is consuming 10-12 calories per pound of bodyweight and adjust accordingly.

Protein consumption post workout is a great option. Many endomorphs will want to stay away from a protein/simple carbohydrate mix, unless the end game is a goal of a higher percentage of body fat.

ENDOMORPH TRAINING TIPS

- Generally perform up to eight sets per body part.
- Majority of reps should be in the 8-15 range.
- Recovery is faster than the mesomorph but slower than the ectomorph.

- Limit carb intake.
- Train with a mixture of steady state cardio and high intensity intervals.

Endomorph Training Frequency Guideline

While endomorphs can train with higher volume and more frequently than mesomorphs, they do not need to train as frequently as ectomorphs. What follows is the number of days of rest recommended for each body part before training it again:

	Days of Rest "Light Day"	Days of Rest "Medium Day"	Days of Rest "Heavy Day"
Large Muscle Groups: • Upper Legs • Lower Back	4	5	6
Medium Size Muscle Groups: • Chest • Upper Back • Biceps • Triceps • Shoulders	3	4	5
Smaller Muscle Groups: • Midsection • Calves • Forearms	2	3	4

MESOMORPH TRAITS

From the moment that his well-proportioned shoulders squeezed into the door frame of the Tijuana Barbell Club, it was obvious that Kirk Peters was a classic mesomorph. Mesomorphs have large bones and defined muscles. Generally, because of the low, narrow waist, they have a tapered V-like torso. Mesomorphs have excellent posture, well-developed arms, and generally have the appearance of broad shoulders and even the fingers can have a muscled-up appearance.

Mesomorphs could very easily be referred to as "easy gainers." Mesomorphs are able to add muscle mass and lose body fat more rapidly than either of the other somatotypes.

MESOMORPH CHALLENGES

Once they begin to train, mesomorphs make great gains regardless of what they do exercise-wise. On the surface this is a blessing, but as one advances, this can be a curse. Since they make easy gains, mesomorphs may develop unsound training practices.

Unsurprisingly, the mesomorph accumulates body fat easier than the ectomorph. When they are young, mesomorphs can generally eat anything and not get fat, but this is not the case as they age. If they want to stay lean or just look good naked, mesomorphs do best with a high protein diet and a moderate carbohydrate and fat intake. Mesomorphs that have gained excessive weight will initially do well with a low carb approach.

Mesomorph Training Tips

- Train with a variety of rep ranges, tempos, and methods.
- Primarily train in the five to eight rep range explosively.
- Muscles take longer to recover—a heavy leg or lower back day can take upward of a week of recovery.
- Train heavy with adequate rest intervals a majority of the time.
- Do cardio up to three times weekly.
- Eat a balanced diet.

Mesomorph Training Frequency Guideline

Of the three body types, mesomorphs need to train the least often. With that in mind, the number of days of rest recommended for each body part before training it again is as follows:

	Days of Rest "Light Day"	Days of Rest "Medium Day"	Days of Rest "Heavy Day"
Large Muscle Groups: • Upper Legs • Lower Back	5	6	7

Medium Size Muscle Groups: • Chest • Upper Back • Biceps • Triceps • Shoulders	4	5	6
Smaller Muscle Groups: • Midsection • Calves • Forearms	3	4	5

CHAPTER THREE
GAS STATION READY
INTERVAL TRAINING

O n the outdoor deck of our gym hung an old beat-up heavy bag. Although the year round beach weather on the central coast of California offers a comfortable climate for outdoor training, it was rare to see gym goers taking their workout outside. With so few people around and the slow creak of a bag turning on its rusted hinges, there was almost a melancholy air sitting over this section of the gym.

It was dusk, and the setting sun cast a pink hue across the sky while we worked some lead jab boxing combinations on the bag. A long shadow preceded Chato as his muscled shoulders filled the doorway to the deck. While normally clad in a cleanly pressed white shirt, on this evening he came outside in a sleeveless tank top that showed his surprisingly muscled arms.

"Nice evening," he said while taking in the natural beauty of the looming night. "What are you boys up to?"

"Working on a combination our boxing coach showed us."

"I see that it works off the jab."

"Yes, it does. You know about boxing?"

"Well, more about fighting than boxing."

"What's the difference?"

"Mexico had legendary great boxers. When I was in Tijuana, I saw the great Vincente Saldiver fight Ismael Laguna in 1964. Later there was Ricardo Lopez from Cuernavaca, and of course, Julio Cesar Chavez. They were all great in the ring, where you fought under Marquess of Queensberry Rules. But I learned about the stuff you want to know when you stumble into an alley behind some kick and stab bar in Ciudad Juarez or if you are pumping gas at 3 a.m. off some lonesome interstate highway.

"For those scenarios, you need a specific type of training and a particular mindset. Charuto refined his training program after working the northern Baja bars for a couple of years. When he first started on the door, he was still kind of skinny. As a hard gainer, it took time for his lifting to show up on his body and bulk out his frame. A tall, skinny kid as the bouncer at rough beer joints in Old Mexico? He fought a lot. Later, when the muscle started to stick to his bones and he got a name that was known from Tijuana to Mexicali, he fought less. But, he never forgot what he learned and he kept training. He even shared some of his secrets with Kirk Peters."

"Why did he teach Kirk Peters?"

"Kirk came from a pretty conventional background. Some sort of prep school upbringing, then off to a prestigious private college and after that he went into the seminary to study theology. Somewhere along the line, he started to feel constricted, confined to a preset path. He wanted to stretch out a little. He wanted to breathe. And Tijuana in the 1960s was the place to do just that.

"He started to train at the Barbell Club and always with a smile. When he found out that Charuto worked the bars, he asked for a job and Charuto give him a try. For some reason, you couldn't say no to Kirk. At the bars, the patrons tested Kirk and he did okay. It seemed he had wrestled some and did a little boxing growing up. But some of them guys didn't play by those rules. So Charuto taught him another way to train."

"What type of training?"

"Interval training that focused less on technique and more on aggression and intensity. In his lesson on fighting is a lesson for living: *You keep swinging and you keep moving forward.*

"When Charuto started to implement this training, he had to make do with what he could scrap together. He couldn't get his hands on a heavy bag—he asked around and none of the local boxing gyms were looking to get rid of a used bag. So he put something together with an old canvas duffel bag that he filled with sand and carpet padding."

Charuto looked off, lost in a memory. "Man, Charuto used to bang on that thing. And somehow, it held up."

Turning toward the heavy bag, Chato ran his weathered hand lightly across its battered surface. His hand skimmed slowly over the hastily laid duct tapped that was meant to cover rips and was doing its job with mediocre efficiency. You could hear the slow scraping of his callused hand on the cracked vinyl. His face appeared calm and peaceful, until his hand stopped and he turned back over his shoulder.

"Let me show you how it works on this bag."

An almost unperceivable spark lit back deep in the narrowed slits of his eyes. In a sharp instant, Chato, who was normally slow like a candle, became a frenzy of directed and efficient movement. Beginning in the hips, his body rotated like a corkscrew and he fired punch after punch into the bag. The sound of hardened flesh and bone connecting with the vinyl made bullet-like cracks that reverberated across the deck and echoed into the gym.

Entranced by the rapid change from placidity to vibrant explosivity, we missed the gym members who were slowly filling the outdoor deck to watch this man work the bag. The first round of this show could not have lasted more than half a minute, but when he stopped for a brief break, we saw that that gym-goers were crowding around to watch this delivery of intensity.

Chato continued on the bag for a number of rounds and we noticed some important details. Technique was not the focus of the drill, but he followed some sound pugilistic movement patterns. When he threw punches, he started with a rotation in the hips that continued across his body. He would not throw "arm punches," or strikes where the power came simply from his upper extremities.

At times, he would move his body to create a new angle of attack. When he did so, he would pivot off his front foot, somewhat similar to a pivot in basketball except that he was sure to stay on his toes. And he would often switch the directions of his pivot. This keeps the potential opponent guessing about which direction the next strike will come from and made Chato more difficult to hit.

Although it was not an overt movement, Chato would rotate the foot on the same side of the punch he was throwing. This rotation was more noticeable when he threw power punches, like hooks and overhand rights.

This is an interval training drill, so you will complete short bursts of intense output followed by brief rest periods. These drills may be done as a finisher on chest days or after shoulder training. They're also a good option for improving general conditioning. Good technique is important for preventing injuries and improving speed and power. However, this drill places an emphasis on movement intensity. During the allotted time, place as many fists on the bag as possible.

In addition to working on a heavy bag, this training also includes a shadow boxing and sprawl drill that should be completed directly after the heavy bag portion of the workout. A sprawl is a movement taken from grappling that prevents a potential takedown. It is performed by squatting and kicking your legs back until you are in a modified push up position (similar to the "Upward Facing Dog" position in yoga, with your hips down and your chest open and facing up), then returning to a standing position.

It is important to drill, or practice, this takedown prevention technique. Whether you find yourself in a back alley in Mexicali or at gas station in the pre-dawn hours, the idea is consistent. You don't want to be taken off your feet and onto the ground, where you can be boot stomped.

Remember that this drill is meant to be performed with complete effort in each round. Greater exertion improves the workout and the direct transference to a self-defense situation.

Week 1
Complete twice during the week.
Heavy Bag Training: Complete eight rounds of 20 seconds with a 20-second break between each round.

- Freestyle punching

Shadow Boxing Training: Complete four rounds of 20 seconds with a 20-second break between each round.

- Throw a four punch combination and sprawl (complete as many times as possible)

Week 2
Complete twice during the week.
Heavy Bag Training: Complete eight rounds of 20 seconds with a 10-second break between each round.

- Freestyle punching

Shadow Boxing Training: Complete four rounds of 20 seconds with a 10-second break between each round.

- Throw a four punch combination and sprawl (complete as many times as possible)

Week 3
Complete three times during the week.
Heavy Bag Training: Complete eight rounds of 30 seconds with a 20-second break between each round.

- Freestyle punching

Shadow Boxing Training: Complete four rounds of 30 seconds with a 20-second break between each round.

- Throw a four punch combination and sprawl (complete as many times as possible)

Week 4
Complete three times during the week.
Heavy Bag Training: Complete eight rounds of 30 seconds with a 10-second break between each round.

- Freestyle punching

Shadow Boxing Training: Complete four rounds of 30 seconds with a 10-second break between each round.

- Throw a four punch combination and sprawl (complete as many times as possible)

CHAPTER FOUR
PAUSE TO BUILD STRENGTH

In the offseason from wrestling and football, we had more time on our hands and spent much of it at the gym, where we focused on building as much muscle as possible for the upcoming year. It was during this time that we were able to make some of our most significant gains. Knowing this, we scoured the gym for as much weight as possible.

On one particular day, we were just getting through our warm up sets on the bench press when we noticed that the majority of the 45 plates were across the gym near a squat rack. Trekking across the gym to find the weights, we left our bench vacant for a moment. Like at many gyms, an empty bench press is a real find and an upscale real estate broker with a bad spray tan gleefully started to load the bar with some 25-pound wheels.

As we walked back with plates in each hand, we saw the interloper, with his trendy workout wear, settling in for his toning presses. We quickened our pace to retrieve our stolen bench. Although we were but teenagers, there was no way that anyone, grown man or not, was getting in the way of our workout.

In no time at all, we confronted the dude, explained the situation, and he was all too happy to be on his way. Across the gym, Chato, resting his thick forearms on the dip bar, quietly took in the state of affairs. With a drop of his head, an easy smile, and a slight headshake, Chato seemed to enjoy seeing the yuppie lifter getting "checked" by a couple of kids.

After it was clear that we were finished with our sets, Chato sauntered over.

"I like how you boys handled yourselves. The bench was yours and you made that clear."

"You can't let too many things get in the way of training," we replied with a youthful confidence in the legitimacy of our statement.

"That's exactly right!" His eyes sparked in enthusiastic agreement and his scarred face widening into a handsome grin.

"But you know," Chato continued, "that's not the only way to do things on the bench press."

"What do you mean?"

"I'll tell you. You see, Charuto invested a lot of time and money into the Tijuana Barbell Club, but he still was low on equipment. For instance, as he got stronger on the bench, he did not always have the plates he needed for heavy lifting. Maybe Oso was using some weight over on the squat rack or Kirk Peters had the bar loaded up for overhead presses. Charuto didn't want to wait for them to finish or go chasing loose plates around the gym.

"Instead he found a method of staying on the bench and banging out more volume, with less weight, and in a shorter time. *Sometimes the best thing to do is pause, take stock of where you are, and make the most of what you have.*

"With this training routine you rarely leave the bench and you make the most of the weight by taking shorter breaks between sets. Many years after I learned about this from Charuto, I talked with some cons who lifted heavy pig iron in the yard of the San Quentin Correctional Facility during the 1970s. They said this was a method common among the strongest convicts and was favorite of Tookie Williams."

"The old school Crip? We saw something about him on some gang documentaries."

"Yes, that's him. A lot of cons liked this training method because you don't have to get up and risk losing your bench. Also, the stronger guys could get a workout with the limited amount of iron that was on yard. Here, let me show you how it works."

Rest-Pause Training Explained
Rest-pause training breaks down one set into several sub-sets with a brief rest between each. Select your chosen exercise and load a weight you can perform for 6–10 repetitions. Lift the weight for as many reps as possible, take a 20 second rest interval, and do the same weight again; this will probably be two to three repetitions. Repeat this process twice, for a total of three sub sets.

If you select the bench press as your exercise, a rest-pause series might look something like this:

Set 1: 250 x 8 reps

Rest 20 seconds

Set 2: 250 x 3 reps

Rest 20 seconds

Set 3: 250 x 2 reps

This method is a great way to bust through a plateau and teach you to grind out reps. Your muscle fibers will be very fatigued and, because of the repetitive bouts with limited rest, you will experience a t-shirt tearing pump.

Since this method is taxing on the central nervous system (CNS), do not use it every workout for every set. Due to the strain imposed on the CNS, avoid doing this method for highly technical movements.

HOW TO USE REST-PAUSE METHODS

» **Determine your purpose:** For strength, generally use 85+ percent; for size, use 70-85 percent; and for muscle endurance, use less than 70 percent. Rest pauses work for all three.

»**Rest Intervals Between Subsets:** Strength 20-60 seconds, size-20-30 seconds, muscle endurance 10-20 seconds.

» **Have Spotter Monitor Rest Periods**: You need to worry about lifting the weight.

»When in Doubt, Stop: We are measuring reps for the duration of three subsets. If the last rep of a set of bench press was an all-out grinder, you will perform poorly on subsequent sets and reduce total rep count. Keep rep records. Rest pausing is the ultimate form of density training, or in other words, getting more done in less time.

Benefits of Rest-Pause Training

Regardless of your genetics, rest pause training has a no-discrimination policy when it comes to making gains. Fast gainers and slow gainers both thrive on it. Unlike traditional single repetition rest pauses that old-time strength athletes swear by, open ended rest pause training allows the athlete to adapt the weight to his individual capabilities. A primarily slow-twitch fiber lifter will get more reps; a fast-twitch lifter will get fewer reps. The bottom line is, both are performing sets at maximum intensity which will prompt strength gains.

While most linear progression schemes have no way to account for auto regulation (that is, the degree of readiness, intensity, and focus that you bring to a particular workout session), rest pausing allows you to continuously and progressively overload your training regardless of the periodization scheme. When utilized correctly, rest pauses are a game changer.

Kirk Peters' Plateau-Busting Chest Routine

The rest-pause method may be applied to a number of different programs and routines. In the storied past of the Tijuana Barbell Club, there were plenty of times the rest pause method broke through training plateaus.

When Kirk first arrived in Old Mexico, he had a beautiful build from his scholastic sports background. Years of lacrosse, wresting, and football left an imprint on Kirk's torso. Although not one to focus on aesthetics, his shoulders were broad and his back was wide from the pulling and clinching in grappling. He was lean from running up and down the field. However, when he turned to the side, his profile showed that his chest was lacking.

Above all else, Kirk believed in balance in life and he wanted that balance to be evident in the body he was building inside of the Tijuana Barbell Club. So he asked Charuto to construct a program that would give him a chest to match the rest of his physique. Charuto used rest-pause training as a central feature in the following workout.

Exercise	Rest Interval	Intensity	Sets	Reps
*Bench Press	20 seconds	85%	Max	2
**Incline Press	20 seconds	80%	Max	2
***Dips	120 seconds	8 rep max	2	6, Max
****Incline Cable Flyes	60 seconds	Max	2	15
*****Dumbbell Pull-over	90 seconds	Moderate	2	20

*Do as many sets of two as possible. If you miss a set of two, stop the exercise and progress to the next movement. If you reach the sixth set, perform as many reps as possible. For all other sets, hit the specified reps.

** Do as many sets of two as possible. If you miss a set of two, stop the exercise and progress to the next movement. If you reach the sixth set, perform as many reps as possible. For all other sets, hit the specified reps.

***Add weight if applicable, and use a forward lean to emphasize working the chest.

****Dumbbells or chains can be substituted if cables are not available.

*****Emphasize the stretch, not the weight used.

CHARUTO'S BULGING BACK ARMS AND BICEPS ROUTINE
Long before Charuto was the legendary bouncer and strongman of 1960s Tijuana, he was a street urchin roaming the back alleys of Old Mexico. But the moment he saw the doorman working the entrance to a trendy night club, he knew that he could, and would, improve his plight in life. As Charuto remembered it, the doorman had a neon light raining down on his head which looked almost like a halo and gave the bouncer an angelic quality. Like a celestial messenger, this bouncer that

Charuto saw as a child was a beacon directing him on his life path.

When he finally took his place at the door of the bars of Tijuana, Charuto wanted to do a good job. One of the first places he worked was the bar inside of Hotel Nelson. Built in 1948 with the first elevator in northwest Mexico and telephones in every room, the hotel was a destination for upscale clients. It is said that many celebrities (like Marilyn Monroe) visited the hotel and its bar. To accommodate the swanky patrons, bouncers at Bar Nelson would often dress up.

When Charuto first got the job, he could not yet afford a nice blazer, or even a long sleeve shirt. But, they gave him a bow tie to wear and he found an old polo shirt that someone left in the hotel lobby. The shirt sleeves were too big for his arms. There was Charuto in an oversized polo shirt, with a black bow tied haphazardly tied around his neck. To make the shirt look better, Charuto realized that he needed to add some bulk to his arms. And he needed to do so quickly.

He created a rest-pause workout similar to this one as a means to solve the issue.

Exercise	Rest Interval	Intensity	Sets	Reps
*Close Grip Bench Press	180 seconds	80%,70%	2	Max
**Incline Hammer Curls		Max	2	15

***EZ Curl French Press	120 seconds	12 rep max	2	10, Max
****Curls		10 rep max	2	8, Max
*****Dumbbell Floor Pause Triceps Extensions	45 seconds	Max	5	8
******Reverse Curls		Max	5	8

*Using a grip approximately two inches closer than your regular bench press, with prescribed percentages of your regular bench press one-repetition max/one rep maximum. For Set 1 do the maximum numbers of reps with 80 percent of your one rep maximum, stopping one rep short of failure. After resting 20 seconds, use the same weight (80 percent of your one rep maximum) and lift it again for a maximum number of reps stopping one short of failure. After resting 20 seconds, finally repeat this a third time. All three mini sets described are one rest-pause set. Refer to this description for rest-pause in subsequent routines. For set two, do the same thing with 70 percent of your max.

**Use approximately a 45-degree incline, keep form strict, and superset with Close Grip Bench Press.

***Keep elbows in and focus on using a full range of motion, emphasizing a comfortable stretch at the bottom of the movement. If you do not have an EZ curl bar, or it causes discomfort, you can substitute a triceps rope or a dumbbell.

****Superset with French press. A barbell or EZ curl can be used and if neither is available, or they cause discomfort, you can use a machine or dumbbells. Set 1 is performed for eight reps. Set 2 uses the same weight but is performed in the rest-pause style described above.

*****If dumbbells are not available, a barbell or EZ curl bar can be substituted. Keep elbows in tight and pause each rep for half a second on the floor.

******To make this exercise more difficult (which is recommended), do it with a fat bar or fat gripz. Superset reverse curls with dumbbell floor triceps extensions.

BIG WHEELS ROLLING LEG ROUTINE

Night after night, Charuto worked the door at many of Tijuana's most popular night spots and he acquired quite a reputation. Sometimes, an aspiring tough guy would show up at the bar, looking to challenge Charuto. A few of these challenges became some of the most legendary feuds in Tijuana lore.

One night, a man came around asking about Charuto. Rather than looking for a fight, Sugar Murray had a business proposition for Charuto. A consummate salesman and hustler, Murray came to Old Mexico from West Los Angeles under the pretense of selling some real estate. But really, he was interested in making some dough by any means necessary. When he heard stories about Charuto, he heard about his strength and his way with the ladies, and he heard that he had what you call charisma.

Once Murray found Charuto, he sold him on extending his growing reputation into a travelling strongman show. Like most things in his life, Charuto wanted to do the best possible job at being a strongman. He understood that he would need more leg strength for many of the strongman feats. To develop his legs, Charuto devised a leg routine using the rest-pause principle.

Exercise	Rest Interval	Intensity	Sets	Reps
*Squats	180 seconds	10 rep max	5	5, 5, 5, 5, max
**Bulgarian Dumbbell Split Squats	90 seconds	Max	3	10, 8, 6
***Leg Press	120 seconds	20 rep max, 15 rep max	2	max
****Leg Curls	90 seconds	max	3	6, 6, Max
*****Dumbbell One Leg RDL	60 seconds	6 rep max	3	6

*Do the last set in a rest-pause style. Front squats or trap bar deadlifts may be used as substitutes.

**Use a full range of motion and a barbell may be substituted.

***Both sets performed in a rest-pause style.

****Use the same weight on set 3 as set 2, but perform set 3 in a rest-pause style.

*****A barbell maybe substituted.

CHARUTO'S STRONG BACK EQUALS STRONG MAN ROUTINE

Many times in the bar, the alleys behind the bar, and the streets in front of the bar, Charuto would be squaring off with power drinkers, belligerent tourists, and local thugs. The murky darkness of the Tijuana night life is home to some of the nastiest types of fighting.

Real functional strength is a valuable tool in these situations. Whether you are peeling a knife from the hands of a member of the local thieves' guild or clinched up against a brick wall trading body blows with two bulked-up Midwestern cornhuskers who let their Mexican vacation get the better of their social inhibitions, you want to develop strength in your posterior chain, or the backside of your body.

The movements necessary for survival in any real combat situation require strength generated from your back. Use this rest-pause workout to build that strength.

Exercise	Rest Interval	Intensity	Sets	Reps
*Deadlifts	120 seconds	6 rep max	6	3
**Dumbbell Shrugs	90 seconds	Max	3	12, 10, 8
***Seal Rows	120 seconds	10 rep max	3	5, 5, Max
****Neutral Grip Pull-ups	180 seconds	max	3	6, 6, Max
*****Seated Rows	30 seconds	15 rep max	8	8

*Assuming you are able to keep good form, snatch grip or deficit deadlifts (no more than a three-inch deficit) may be substitutes.

**Hold each repetition in the top contracted position for three seconds. If dumbbells are not available, a barbell, hammer strength machine or hise shrugs on a calf raise machine may be substitutes.

***Dumbbells or a neutral grip barbell or a chest supported row machine may substitutes. Use the same weight on all three sets, and do the third set in the rest-pause style described above.

****Go as heavy as possible on the first two sets by adding additional weight if applicable. Band assistance can be used if you are unable to use bodyweight. Use the same weight on the third set as on the second but do it in the rest-pause style.

*****Do the final set in a rest-pause style.

Oso's Male Stripper Shoulder Routine
(aka#OLDSCHOOLBLOODANDGUTSMALESTRIPPER)

The first member of Charuto's Tijuana Barbell Club was the large ursine looking lifter, Oso. Wide and broad with a thick pelt of hair, Oso resembled the iconic, but now extinct, California Grizzly. With this broad build, Oso was a menacing presence at the door of the Tijuana bars he worked.

Most nights, Oso worked alongside Charuto at the Tijuana night spots. Without fail, he had Charuto's back in some of the stickiest situations. Acting as Charuto's closest confidant and ally was all that Oso wanted, until he came up with the idea of male stripping for the wealthy tourist girls who came to vacation in Old Mexico.

To make this dream a reality, Oso needed to harden up his body. Charuto was never one to stand in the way of a friend's dream, no matter how unusual it may sound. To help Oso, Charuto put together a rest-pause workout to build a set of shoulders that would make ladies swoon in passionate desire and men sigh in jealousy.

Exercise	Rest Interval	Intensity	Sets	Reps
*Face Pulls	120 seconds	Maximum	3	12
**Incline Face Down Rear Swings 6 Inch Range of Motion		Maximum	3	25
***Bent Over Fly		Maximum	3	6
****Overhead Press	180 seconds	8 Rep Max	6	3
*****Seated Lateral Raise	60 seconds	8 rep max, 12 rep max, 15 rep max	3	max

*A band or a cable can be used. Hold the contraction for one second, while purposefully focusing on the contraction in the posterior deltoids.

**Using momentum, swing the dumbbells facedown for a six inch range of motion. Go as heavy as possible, while purposefully focusing all intention on the posterior deltoids doing the work (great video example on the Jailhouse Strong YouTube).

***Hold the contracted position for one second and use a three second negative to further enhance mind muscle connection on the posterior deltoids. Face pulls, rear delt swings, and bent over fly are all one large giant set.

TIJUANA BARBELL CLUB REST-PAUSE LIMIT STRENGTH PROGRAM

When Chato explained the Tijuana Barbell Club style of rest-pause training he emphasized that this program places a fair amount of stress on the body. In particular, the lifter who is new to the iron may not have the base level of muscular structure to successfully navigate a true rest-pause workout. With this in mind, he recommended using this more approachable type of the rest-pause method to build a base level of strength, which will pre-pare the lifter for more extreme and intense measures.

The rest-pause limit strength program is laid out in four-week cycles that can be followed easily. This program is meant to accomplish two things. First, this workout is designed to increase your limit, or foundational, strength. With a solid base of limit strength, you can develop your functional training and more explosive movements.

Second, some novice lifters may find that rest-pause training is a bit difficult initially. This pro-gram offers a more accessible entry into the strenu-ous nature of rest-pause training.

For supplementary and assistance exercises, pick from the list below, but remember to follow the specified rep protocols. All supplementary and assistance movements should be completed as heavy as possible, stopping just shy of muscle failure or technical breakdown of the movement.

You have the freedom to make the program fit your individual specifications with auxiliary and assistance work. Everyone has different sticking points and requirements, so use the supplemental training that works best for you. Each time you repeat a supplemental exercise, strive to pile a little more pig iron on the bar, even if it is just a couple of pounds.

On the last set of a core movement, if the weight feels good, do it in a rest-pause format. This means that you will do it for as many reps as possible while maintaining great technique. If your form breaks down, terminate the set. After your first set is complete, rest 20 seconds and do the same thing for a second time (assuming that your technique is optimal). After the second set, rest 20 seconds and do it a third time. In this way, a rest-pause set is really three mini-sets. Remember, stop if your technique is compromised.

Never go heavy during the deload week, because this is when active recovery allows for the largest strength gains to take place.

After a four-week cycle is complete (three weeks of buildup training and the one-week deload), start over. At the beginning of each four-week cycle, add five pounds to each core lift; or if you feel ambitious, add 10 pounds. Never more!

After the deload week, your body is fresh and rested. This is an ideal time to achieve a new personal record or max out. You can retest your maximum lifts after three four-week cycles. If these jumps seem small, then lift the weight more explosively and do more reps! You will get stronger.

Frequency

A requisite level of recovery is a foundational aspect of this program. So always rest at least 48 hours between workouts. On paper, this program appears to be three days a week. However, remember that the seven-day week is a man-made concept; it has nothing to do with physiology, or how you adapt to training.

If you cannot train three days a week, make your workout week 8-10 days, because this is your program! In the same light, if you recover well, you can condense your work week to six days, but never shorter than five days.

In a nutshell, the idea is to complete the week and then add five pounds to the core lift each time you perform the rep scheme each four-week cycle. If the weight is light, do it more explosively, and do more repetitions on your rest-pause set. This program can be done for many successive months, if you are disciplined and do not add excessive weight.

Remember, the core lifts are the key. So follow the prescribed exercises and weights. But we encourage you to switch supplementary and assistance exercises.

THE PROGRAM

Week 1

Day 1

Exercise	Intensity	Sets	Reps
Squats	65%, 75%, 80%	3	10, 8, 5
Lower Body Supplementary		3	
Lower Body Assistance Superset Hamstring/ Your Choice		3	
Heavy Neck		3	
Abdominal		3	

Day 2

Exercise	Intensity	Sets	Reps
Bench Press	65%, 75%, 80%	3	10, 8, 5
Upper Body Supplementary		3	
Upper Assistance Superset Bicep/Tricep		3	
Light Neck		3	
Pull-ups (Any Grip)		3	Max

Day 3

Exercise	Intensity	Sets	Reps
Deadlift	75%	3	5
Upper Body Supplementary		3	
Lower Body Supplementary		3	
Full body Supplementary		3	
Full Body Assistance/ Superset Heavy Neck		3	

Week 2

Day 1

Exercise	Intensity	Sets	Reps
Squats	65%, 75%, 85%	3	3
Lower Body Supplementary		3	
Lower Body Assistance Superset Hamstring/ Your Choice		3	
Heavy Neck		3	
Abdominal		3	

Day 2

Exercise	Intensity	Sets	Reps
Bench Press	65%, 75%, 85%	3	3
Upper Body Supplementary		3	
Upper Assistance Superset Bicep/Triceps		3	
Light Neck		3	
Pull-ups (Any Grip)		3	Max

Day 3

Exercise	Intensity	Sets	Reps
Deadlift	65%, 75%, 85%	3	3
Upper Body Supplementary		3	
Lower Body Supplementary		3	
Full Body Supplementary		3	
Full Body Assistance/ Superset Heavy Neck		3	

Week 3
Day 1

Exercise	Intensity	Sets	Reps
Squats	70%, 75%, 80%, 85%, 90%	5	5, 4, 3, 2, 1
Lower Body Supplementary		3	
Lower Body Assistance Superset Hamstring/ Your Choice		3	
Heavy Neck		3	
Abdominal		3	

Day 2

Exercise	Intensity	Sets	Reps
Bench Press	70%, 75%, 80%, 85%, 90%	5	5, 4, 3, 2, 1
Upper Body Supplementary		3	
Upper Assistance Superset Bicep/Triceps		3	
Light Neck		3	
Pull-ups (Any Grip)		3	

Day 3

Exercise	Intensity	Sets	Reps
Deadlift	70%, 75%, 80%, 85%, 90%	5	5, 4, 3, 2, 1
Upper Body Supplementary		3	
Lower Body Supplementary		3	
Full Body Supplementary		3	
Full Body Assistance/ Superset Heavy Neck		3	

Week 4 (Deload)

Day 1

Exercise	Intensity	Sets	Reps
Squats	70%	5	2
Lower Body Supplementary	70%	2	
Lower Body Assistance Superset Hamstring/ Your Choice	70%	2	
Heavy Neck	70%	2	
Abdominal		3	

Day 2

Exercise	Intensity	Sets	Reps
Bench Press	70%	5	2
Upper Body Supplementary	70%	2	
Upper Assistance Superset Bicep/Tricep	70%	2	
Light Neck	70%	2	
Pull-ups (Any Grip)	70%	1	Max

Day 3

Exercise	Intensity	Sets	Reps
Deadlift	70%	2	3
Upper Body Supplementary	70%	2	
Lower Body Supplementary	70%	2	
Full Body Supplementary	70%	2	
Full Body Assistance/ Superset Heavy Neck	70%	2	

CHAPTER FIVE
WATCHING WAVES AND
BUILDING SETS

If you were an adolescent male who spent hours hitting the pig iron, sometimes it was nice to be noticed for your work. Growing up along the southern coast of California, a year-round Mediterranean climate meant that the beach remained a consistent recreational option and it was just the place to be spotted by the young girls who spread out their towels along the miles of soft sand that stretched down to the sea coves.

We trained more for function than form and we wanted go-muscles, not show-muscles. The result was a body composition that was more dense than defined, but still a torso that we displayed proudly on a sunny beach day.

While strolling down the beach one day, we noticed the building swell and saw more and more surfers working their way down to the water with the intent of making the most of the waves. Along the water, disparate groups gathered in different sections of the beach. Far from the building surf, you had some sort of a family reunion coming together with an array of potato chips and soft drinks being passed around. Down farther along the beach, there were steep cliffs that built in size as they jutted out toward the point of the cove. Under the relative cover of the cliff face was a party crowd tapping a small keg and playing rock music on a boom box. Scattered in between were small groups of girls and guys making the most of the pleasant weather.

Out at the end of the point, where the land protruded toward the section of the water where the waves peaked and broke, a lone figure sat. As we walked closer, we got a better look at the solitary beachcomber and recognized our conversation partner, Chato, from the gym. With the sun at our back, our shadows reached Chato before we did, and feeling the shadow falling across his broad shoulders, he turned with squinting eyes to meet our gaze.

"Hey boys, nice day. Any luck with the girls?"

We chuckled and mumbled a somewhat incoherent adolescent response.

Despite all of the time that we talked with Chato, we still felt a little nervous around him, partially because we were slightly in awe of him. Plus this was the first time we saw him out of the context of the gym. Although he stood out at the fitness center, he still could be placed alongside other lifters because of his build. However, at the beach where families gathered, yuppies picnicked, and girls in trendy bikinis applied glistening layers of suntan lotion, he seemed anachronistic, or somewhat outdated. His rough features and leathery skin made it seem like he stepped out of an old western movie onto a modern day beach setting.

"Well, girls or not, it is nice to come to the beach and sit by the water. When I first met Charuto, it was on a day like this and he was sitting along the ocean."

"How did you meet Charuto?"

"My family had just moved from Bahia de Kino along the Sea of Cortez in Sonora. My mom got a job cleaning hotel rooms and my dad worked as a mechanic. He could fix just about anything on wheels."

Chato turned to the horizon and paused after mentioning his parents, before turning back to us.

"That meant that I had long empty days to myself. My first week in Tijuana, I was walking along the beach and I saw this tall, gallant gentleman sitting and staring out at the ocean. It was Charuto. He noticed me looking at him and invited me to train at his gym. I was just a scrawny kid, but under his tutelage I filled out. If it wasn't for Charuto, I don't know what would have happened to me.

"You know," Chato continued, "there are some good waves around northern Baja and Charuto would watch the surf for hours. He learned a lot from watching the sets rolling in."

"What did he learn?"

"He learned about patience and commitment."

"What do you mean?"

"Okay, see the surfers out there?" Chato asked while pointing out to the nearby surf break in the ocean.

"Yes, where they are all gathered together, like in a group?"

"They only seem like they are one group. Wait, and watch what happens when the next set, or series of waves, comes through."

So, we took a seat alongside Chato to wait and to watch.

In a short time, a good size wave built and rolled toward the shore. A number of the younger surfers paddled frantically to make this first wave. A couple of surfers made the wave. However, a second bigger wave emerged from behind the first with an older crew taking off on this wave. Finally, the last wave of the set appeared. It was clearly the biggest and the lone surfer who took this wave was obviously the most experienced. As for the surfers who went for the first wave, they were stuck in the inside impact zone and were hit with the full power of heavy second and third waves.

The veteran surfers who took the later waves were able to calmly paddle back out to the top of the line up without taking a beating from the later waves in the set.

We told Chato what we witnessed.

"Good eye," Chato said. "You see," he continued, "the experienced veteran has learned to not take off on, or put all his strength into, the first wave unless he has the strength to endure the entire set.

"Take a look around this beach. See them pretty boys over there?" Chato asked as he lifted his chin in the direction of some frat boys from the local university who gathered around a few attractive coeds. With their loud neon swim trunks, the frat boys were hard to miss.

We nodded in response.

So Chato continued. "At first glance they appear strong. Some form in the biceps and slight ripples in the abs. But, look at their back and up through their shoulders. There is no density, no depth of strength.

"Charuto used to put us through something called wave loading. Kids like that would go all out on the first wave of the training and, like the young surfers you just watched, they would get hammered by the second and third waves. You want the type of physique that consists of muscles that respond readily to the increase in the load or obstacle. *Real strength builds with the challenge.* Wave training builds that kind of durable strength."

"What is wave loading?" we asked.

"I will explain it."

WAVE LOADING OVERVIEW
Wave Loading is a method used to increasingly stimulate the nervous system. Each wave consists of three

sets, and since we are training maximal strength in the bench press, we will keep the reps to three or fewer. A traditional wave for someone who bench presses 300 pounds will look like this.

Warm-Up

Set	Rest Interval	Weight	Reps
1	30 seconds	Bar	10
2	30 seconds	Bar	10
3	60 seconds	135	6
4	90 seconds	185	4
5	120 seconds	225	3
6	120 seconds	255	1
7	150 seconds	285	1

Wave 1

Set	Rest Interval	Weight	Reps
1	3-5 Minutes	270	3
2	3-5 Minutes	285	2
3	3-5 Minutes	300	1

Wave 2

Set	Rest Interval	Weight	Reps
1	3-5 Minutes	275	3
2	3-5 Minutes	290	2
3	3-5 Minutes	305	1

Each wave would call for an additional five pounds to be added for each set. Many athletes will get through two waves the first time they attempt this workout; some gifted athletes may hit four waves or more. Some programs call for the athlete to cease at four waves; others call for continuous waves until failure by following the same progression.

WHY IT WORKS

Here is the Cliffs Notes version of why it works:

Wave loading is based on the principal of post-tetanic facilitation. The earlier sets prepare the central nervous system and work muscles so they are able to contract with greater amounts of force, or lift more weight on the later sets.

The top single in a wave will cause the following wave to seem easier. The first wave prepares you for the next wave. With this in mind, realize that the first wave may be the most difficult because it is not preceded by a preparatory wave.

THE PROGRAM

In the wave program described below, stop before you hit failure. REPEAT, DO NOT MISS REPS! If you plan to run this program weekly, do not exceed four waves—no matter what. Someone who is running this program monthly, or less frequently, would do as many waves possible.

Wave Loading Bench Press Program
Wave 1

Set	Rest Interval	Weight	Reps
1	3-5 Minutes	86%	3
2	3-5 Minutes	91%	2
3	3-5 Minutes	96%	1

Wave 2

Set	Rest Interval	Weight	Reps
1	3-5 Minutes	88%	3
2	3-5 Minutes	93%	2
3	3-5 Minutes	98%	1

Wave 3

Set	Rest Interval	Weight	Reps
1	3-5 Minutes	90%	3
2	3-5 Minutes	95%	2
3	3-5 Minutes	100%	1

Wave 4

Set	Rest Interval	Weight	Reps
1	3-5 Minutes	92%	3
2	3-5 Minutes	97%	2
3	3-5 Minutes	102%	1

Accessory Exercises

Pick one accessory exercise from each group listed below and perform it in the prescribed rep range. If you completed one or two waves, you will complete three to fout sets of any one exercise from Group 1, Group 2, and Group 3. If you completed three waves, you will complete two to three sets of any one exercise from each of the three groups. If you completed four waves, you will complete one to two sets of any one exercise from each of the three groups.

Group 1 (4-6 Rep Range) Dips, Close Grip Bench Press, Spoto Press

Group 2 (6-8 Rep Range) Dumbbell Pause Bench Press, Incline Press Any Variation, Floor Press

Group 3 (10-15 Range) Any Triceps Ext Variation, Dips, Any Triceps Pushdown Variation

Further Guidelines

- All bench presses during the concentric phase must be performed as explosively as possible.
- Do not perform this program more than once a week, but a second lighter accessory day is fine.
- Completing two waves or more calls for a two percent increase in the following

weeks' starting weights. If you do not hit at least two waves, do not progress in weight.

- Never miss a rep.
- This program can be run sporadically to shake things up (once monthly works great, while keeping with the same progression).
- This program should not be run weekly more than seven weeks straight (you must complete a deload during Week 4).
- For the accessory work, target weakness and keep in mind everything that is subservient to the bench press.

Sample Deload Week
Exercises/Sets/Reps
*Bench Press/3/6
**Group 1/2/5
***Group 2/2/8
****Group 3/2/10

Exercise Notes
*Use 65-70% of your max for all three sets.
**Use 70% of the weight you are capable of for five reps.
*** Use 70% of the weight you are capable of for eight reps.
**** Use 70% of the weight you are capable of for 10 reps.
*****These guidelines can serve as the second optional bench press day.

*****For each selected group, pick only one exercise per group just like the wave loading workouts.

Wave Loading Squat Program
Wave 1

Set	Rest Interval	Weight	Reps
1	4-6 Minutes	82%	3
2	4-6 Minutes	89%	2
3	4-6 Minutes	96%	1

Wave 2

Set	Rest Interval	Weight	Reps
1	4-6 Minutes	86%	3
2	4-6 Minutes	91%	2
3	4-6 Minutes	98%	1

Wave 3

Set	Rest Interval	Weight	Reps
1	4-6 Minutes	92%	3
2	4-6 Minutes	97%	2
3	4-6 Minutes	100%	1

Wave 4

Set	Rest Interval	Weight	Reps
1	4-6 Minutes	94%	3
2	4-6 Minutes	99%	2
3	4-6 Minutes	102%	1

ACCESSORY EXERCISES

Pick one accessory exercise from each group listed below and perform it in the prescribed rep range. If you completed one or two waves, you will complete two to three sets of any one exercise from Group 1, Group 2, and Group 3. If you completed three waves, you will complete one to two sets of any one exercise from each of the three groups. If you completed four waves, you will complete one set of any one exercise from each of the three groups.

Group 1 (2-4 Rep Range) Pause Squats, Olympic Pause Squats, Front Squats

Group 2 (6-8 Rep Range) Glute Ham Raises, Olympic Squats, Leg Curls

Group 3 (10-15 Range) Dead Stop Leg Presses, Belt Squats, Sled Drags 20 Yards

FURTHER GUIDELINES

- All squats during the concentric phase must be performed as explosively as possible.
- Do not perform this program more than once a week, but a second lighter accessory day is fine.
- Completing two waves or more calls for a two percent increase in the following weeks' starting weights. If you do not hit at least two waves, do not progress in weight.

- Never miss a rep.
- This program can be run sporadically to shake things up (once monthly works great, while keeping with same progression).
- This program should not be run weekly more than eight weeks straight (you must complete a deload during Weeks 3 and 5; most people do best with five weeks).
- For the accessory work, target weakness and keep in mind that everything is subservient to the squat.

Sample Deload Week
Exercise/Sets/Reps
*Squat/3/5
**Group 1/2/3
***Group 2/2/5
****Group 3/2/10

Exercise Notes
*Use 65-70 percent of your max for all three sets.
**Use 70 percent of the weight you are capable of for three reps.
*** Use 70 percent of the weight you are capable of for five reps.
**** Use 70 percent of the weight you are capable of for 10 reps.
*****These guidelines can serve as the second optional squat day.
******Sled Drags are performed backwards to target the quads.

******* For each selected group, pick only one exercise per group just like the wave loading workouts.

WAVE LOADING DEADLIFT PROGRAM
Wave 1

Set	Rest Interval	Weight	Reps
1	4-6 Minutes	82%	3
2	4-6 Minutes	89%	2
3	4-6 Minutes	96%	1

Wave 2

Set	Rest Interval	Weight	Reps
1	4-6 Minutes	86%	3
2	4-6 Minutes	91%	2
3	4-6 Minutes	98%	1

Wave 3

Set	Rest Interval	Weight	Reps
1	4-6 Minutes	92%	3
2	4-6 Minutes	97%	2
3	4-6 Minutes	100%	1

Wave 4

Set	Rest Interval	Weight	Reps
1	4-6 Minutes	94%	3
2	4-6 Minutes	99%	2
3	4-6 Minutes	102%	1

Accessory Exercises

Pick one accessory exercise from each group listed below and perform it in the prescribed rep range. If you completed one to two waves, you will complete two to three sets of any one exercise from Group 1, Group 2, and Group 3. If you completed three waves, you will complete one to two sets of any one exercise from each of the three groups. If you completed four waves, you will complete one set of any one exercise from each of the three groups.

Group 1 (2-4 Rep Range) Deficit Deadlifts (three inches or less), Romanian Deadlifts, Rack Pulls

Group 2 (6-8 Rep Range) Glute Ham Raises, Barbell Hip Thrust, Bent Over Rows

Group 3 (10-15 Range) Shrugs, Seal Rows, Weighted Back Extensions

Further Guidelines

- All deadlifts must be performed as explosively as possible.
- Do not perform this program more than once a week—NO LIGHTER DAY ALLOWED.
- Completing two waves or more calls for a two percent increase in the following weeks' starting weights. If you do not hit at least two waves, do not progress weights.

- Never miss a rep.
- This program can be run sporadically to shake things up (once monthly works great, while keeping with same progression).
- This program should not be run weekly more than eight weeks straight (you must complete a deload every other week, Example Week 1-Wave Load, Week 2-Deload, Week 3-Wave Load, Week 4-Deload, repeat this sequence for eight weeks).
- For the accessory work, target weakness and keep in mind everything that is subservient to the deadlift.

Sample Deload Week
Exercise/Sets/Reps
*Squat/5/1
**Group 1/2/5
***Group 2/2/6
****Group 3/2/10

Exercise Notes
*Use 65-70 percent of your max for all five sets
**Use 70 percent of the weight you are capable of for five reps
*** Use 70 percent of the weight you are capable of for six reps
**** Use 70 percent of the weight you are capable of for 10 reps
***** For each selected group pick only one exercise per group just like the wave loading workouts.

CHAPTER SIX
THE SHOCK METHOD
CHALLENGE

We spoke frequently with Chato and gained many insights into the old-time training practices favored by Charuto and the crew at the Tijuana Barbell Club. We learned about the ways in which we could apply these training procedures to our workout program.

Eventually, it dawned on us that we were receiving all of this wisdom from Chato because he was a constant presence at the gym. Other folks that we knew from the gym would be there intermittently and while inside the house of iron, they would frequently waste time. In contrast, aside from passing along pearls of wisdom to us (his receptive audience), Chato filled his gym time with a seeming whirlwind of working weights.

Although young and relative newcomers to the iron game, we already were familiar with the notion of overtraining and the law of diminishing returns. With this in mind, we asked Chato as much.

"After I met Charuto on the beach, he took me into the Tijuana Barbell and under his wing. But first, he tested me. It was the same treatment for all new Tijuana Barbell members. It was a physical challenge, but it was also a lesson in mental durability. The basic lesson applies to life and training. A lot of people respond to a challenge in the gym in a manner similar to the way in which they face an obstacle in life: they may dread it or prolong it and some even attempt to shirk or run from it. In my experience, none of these is beneficial and they do not prove successful.

"So, in the midst of Charuto's shock workout challenge, I came to a realization. *When going through a challenge, the best response is to keep on going.*"

"Why did he test you?"

"For a couple of reasons. First, Charuto wanted to ensure that you had the *tenacidad*…the tenacity… the toughness to stay with the training protocols in place at the Tijuana Barbell Club. The mentality for training back in Old Mexico was different."

With a slight lift of the chin, Chato gestured toward Thomas. He was an amateur bodybuilder who worked as carpenter. But a fair amount of Thomas' time was devoted to setting up sexual rendezvous, an activity in which he was currently engaged as he excitedly cavorted with a young married couple.

In a terse manner, Chato said, "There was none of that in the gym."

And without breaking stride, Chato dropped the side of his head in the direction of Ted, an aspiring mover and shaker in the real estate world. As such, Ted seemed to be consistently looking to close a sale and was doing just that at the moment.

"And none of that," Chato continued as he looked at Ted from the corner of his eye.

"When you came through the arches of the Tijuana Barbell, you came to toil in the endless pursuit of perfection. Although Kirk was in the midst of a respite from his divinity school, he had a knack for weaving together a parable and preaching to the Tijuana Barbell crew about the notion that perfection was unattainable for mere humans. Nonetheless, the pursuit of perfection, in this instance through the iron, was worthy in of itself. In other words, Kirk would explain, the unachievable destination creates a situation where the journey becomes the source of fulfillment.

"Like anything of value in life, training with the iron has only as much meaning as the work you put into the experience. Charuto tested me because he wanted to know that I was able to work hard and to see the value in hard work.

"But Charuto also tested me because it was meant to shock my body into getting stronger. In fact, a central aspect of Charuto's program was shocking your system. It was not for those who lacked *fortaleza*, or fortitude. How you say, internal strength. You needed that to get through this shock method of training. Let me explain how it works."

From the onset, you want to recognize that this is a program solely for the physically and mentally strong lifter. If you fit that description, there are some important ideas to identity with this program. They are as follows:

Distribute Intensity—There will be a minimum of 72 hours between sessions that require eccentric emphasis loads, maximal loads, and going to failure. While the key is a constant stimulus to the muscle we want to grow, during some sessions we will annihilate the working muscles and in other workouts, we will only mildly stimulate them.

Train Different Movements—The likelihood of overtraining decreases when you do not train the same movements every workout. By hitting the muscle at "different angles" we will also insure recruitment of the widest pool of motor units for maximal hypertrophy.

Distribute Volume—Because we are not training 20+ sets per workout, we will recover much more quickly. We will still do more volume over the course of the week, even though we are not doing a high number of sets during each training session.

Contractions—To optimize recovery and results, we will train eccentrically, concentrically, and isometrically.

Holistic Training—Because we are training at a variety of rep ranges and tempos, we will develop the entire muscle fiber, something that is impossible with just training slow or fast, or solely high reps or low reps.

SHOCK TRAINING WORKOUT PROGRAMS

The lifters who frequented the Tijuana Barbell Club in Old Mexico came in all sizes. The *veteranos,* or veterans, of the Tijuana Barbell Club—Oso, Kirk Peters, and Charuto—were clear examples of the three most common body types. Although different in their shape and unique in the way in which they acquired muscle, they shared a common physical feature. As a consequence of the arduous demands of training in the Tijuana Barbell Club style, they all developed a thick layer of dense muscularity which coated the entirety of their body.

In fact, among the physical culture circles in Old Mexico during the 1960s, density, more than size or definition, became the trademark characteristic of the Tijuana Barbell Club. However, there is no shortcut, or easy path, to developing a similar concentration of muscle.

For those who are physically, mentally, and spiritually prepared for Tijuana Barbell Club training, the shock method will develop muscular density.

This is lifting in the old style, so it does not rely on technological advances or the comforts of modernity to ease your experience. The only path to success on this journey is the time, intensity, and energy that you are willing to devote to the unabashed improvement of your physicality.

This program exists on a fine line between hard training and over training. While there is a decrease in complete rest time, physical recovery and growth occurs through the constant distribution in movements, rep ranges, and volume. You should expect to be physically exhausted from this workout program.

SHOCK TRAINING FOR THE CHEST

While Charuto did not lift for aesthetics, he did appreciate the timeless splendor of a muscular physique. When Charuto started lifting, he paid particular attention to his chest. He knew that a barrel chest commanded immediate respect in any *barrio*, or neighborhood, on either side of the border.

Without a genetically muscular body type, Charuto could not simply suggest growth. Rather, he demanded muscular development. A shock training program, like the one detailed below, was Charuto's preferred means for building a massive chest.

Day 1
Exercise Sets/Reps
Bench Press 3/5*
Negative Overload Bench Press 3/5**
Dumbbell Incline Fly 2/6-8***

Starting the week off with heavy, compound lifts will ensure that you are putting the most fast-twitch muscle fiber into play when you are fresh. As the week wears on, bigger weight loads will be more difficult to manage because of Central Nervous System (CNS) fatigue, so it's important to start off with a bang.

Why the negatives? Numerous studies show that for a cascade of reasons ranging from satellite cell proliferation to preferential fast-twitch muscle fiber recruitment, eccentric overload movements are superior for inducing muscle hypertrophy.

*Choose a weight that brings failure at five reps. Do not sandbag; start off as heavy as possible and, if needed, reduce weight with each subsequent set. Rest two to three minutes between sets.

** Use 5-15 percent over your one repetition max. Lower the weight for a steady five second tempo. You can lift more eccentrically, so you will. A spotter will assist you on the concentric—all the work is on the negative, so spotters need to aggressively lift the load from the bottom position. Rest four to five minutes between sets.

*** As heavy as possible; do not sacrifice range of motion for additional weight. Rest 60 seconds between sets.

Day 2
Exercise Sets/Reps
Dumbbell Bench Press 3/20*
Incline Dumbbell Press 3/20*

Eccentrics are superior for muscle building, but this type of contraction takes the longest to recover from because eccentrics cause the most muscle damage and recruit the largest muscle fibers, which take the longest to recover—not to mention being most stressful to the CNS.

We are going light but still stimulating the muscle—this will actually expedite recovery. This strategy is commonly known in athletic circles as "active recovery."

*Use the equivalent of 40 percent of your barbell bench press max. For a person with a 200-pound bench press one rep max, that would be 80 pounds. In other words, perform the exercise with two 40 pound dumbbells. Rest 90 seconds between sets.

**Use 30 percent of one rep max barbell bench press. Rest 90 seconds between sets.

Day 3
Exercise Sets/Reps
Push-ups 5/50% of Max *
Isometric Squeeze 5/15 Seconds **

Because of the extreme muscle damage from Day 1, we are not lifting heavy quite yet. Most gym rats do not take advantage of bodyweight movements. Bodyweight movements take less time to recover from because they are closed kinetic chain movements. In other words, you push yourself through space instead of an external object like a barbell or machine—this is natural, easier on the joints and requires less recovery time.

A recent study showed that practicing isometric bodybuilding poses resulted in a muscle mass increase similar to a weight training regimen. We will take full advantage of this!

*Do 50 percent of the maximum reps you could do for one set. If you can do 30 push-ups, you will be doing sets of 15. Rest two minutes between supersets.

**Immediately after each set of push-ups, bend your arms to 90 degrees while standing and holding hands together, and squeeze the chest as hard as possible for 15 seconds.

Day 4
Exercise Sets/Reps
Reverse Grip Bench Press 3/6-8 *
Reverse Grip Dumbbell Bench Press 2/max in 40 seconds **
Dips 3/5 ***

We are recovered and after two days of stimulation, it's time for annihilation!

Why the reverse grip? A recent Canadian study showed that the reverse grip bench press increased upper chest activation by 30 percent compared to a traditional/flat pronated grip bench press. Comparatively, inclines produce about five percent greater upper pec activation over the traditional bench presses.

*Reach failure between six and eight reps, no sandbagging. Rest two to three minutes between sets.

**Use a weight you can do 10 reps with. Control the weight on the negative and explode on the positive. Upon reaching failure, DO NOT drop the weight. Keep going with partials. Even if you are moving the weight one centimeter, do not drop it. Rest two minutes between sets.

***Lean forward to put emphasis on chest. All of these should be a maximum—if you are strong enough to add additional weight, do so. Rest three minutes between sets.

Day 5
Exercise Sets/Reps
Dumbbell Decline Bench Press 3/20*
Neutral Grip Dumbbell Bench Press 3/20**

Although the exercises are different than Day 2, the rational for sets, reps, and intensity is the same.

*Dumbbell decline bench press use the equivalent of 40 percent of your barbell bench press max.

**Dumbbell neutral grip bench press use 30 percent of one rep max barbell bench press. Rest 90 seconds between sets.

Day 6
Exercise Sets/Reps
Cable Fly 3/8*
Feet Elevated Push-ups 3/20**

Our goal today is the "pump," which is one of the mechanisms that induces hypertrophy.

*Pick a weight that you can use for a full range of motion for 12 reps; failure is not the objective. Hold each rep at the top contracted position for half a second, emphasizing the squeeze. Rest one minute between sets.

**Perform push-ups with feet elevated on a bench. Perform the negative for three seconds and explode through the positive. Rest 90 seconds between sets.

Day 7
Repeat Day 3

SHOCK TRAINING FOR SHOULDERS

When Kirk Peters first walked through the door at the Tijuana Barbell Club, it was like an eclipse swept through the gym as his massive shoulders blocked out any shining sunlight. Someone not familiar with the personality and character of Kirk Peters may assume that he would be content with shoulders like granite boulders.

However, the thing about Kirk Peters is that he constantly chased perfection. As a deeply spiritual man, Kirk realized that while flawlessness is a divine station, humanity may strive for a connection to the highest celestial realm by reaching for that ever-elusive state of perfection that brings one ever closer to a divine vicinity.

As a consequence, Kirk would consistently look for means and methods to broaden, deepen, and thicken his shoulders, which filled the doors of the many bars Kirk worked in *Ciudad Tijuana*. One of Kirk's favorite shoulder routines was a shock method program devised by Charuto and similar to the one described below.

Day 1
Exercise Sets/Reps
Overhead Press 3/5*
Incline Lateral Raise five-second negative**2/5
Face Pull/Hand Stand Push-Up Superset 10/failure***

*Perform these standing, using strict technique. For the first two sets, the weight should be one shy of failure; select a weight you are able to complete six reps with. On the final set, go to failure. Upon failure, stop. Rest two to three minutes between sets.

**Each set is a maximum weight to failure. Make sure to follow the five-second negative and you should feel a stretch at the bottom of the movement. The slow eccentric and the stretch are the primary overload mechanisms not the weight, so do not cheat technique. Rest one to two minutes between sets.

*Feel the rear and side deltoids contract as you perform the face pull. Hold the contracted position for one second. If you cheat during this movement, you will miss many of the benefits. If you are unable to traditional handstand push-ups, give the downward dog variation a shot. Rest two minutes between supersets.

Day 2
Exercise Sets/Reps
Single-arm cable lateral raise* 5/15
The single arm (unilateral work) can help offset potential strength imbalances. The cable provides continuous tension on the movement and it is very joint-friendly.

*You will be in and out of the gym quickly today, hold each rep in the contracted position for half a second, emphasizing the side delt contraction. Use a weight you are capable of doing 20 reps with; these should not be taken to failure. Rest one to two minutes between sets.

Day 3
Overhead Press 5/12 *
Bent Over Lateral Fly 5/12 **

*Use 60 percent of the maximum weight you could do for one set of 12 reps. Rest for one minute between sets.

** Use 60 percent of the maximum weight you could do for one set of 12 reps. Hold the contracted position for half a second. Rest for one minute between sets.

Day 4
Exercise Sets/Reps
Ahrens Press 3/6-8 *
Lean Away Dumbbell Lateral Raise 3/12**
Savickas Press 3/3 ***

The Ahrens Press and Lean Away Dumbbell Lateral Raise are a superset; both exercises should be done as heavy as possible.

*Perform Ahrens Press by completing the following steps:

1. Grasp two dumbbells and lift them to shoulder level with a pronated grip.
2. From shoulder position, press the dumbbells out laterally (away from you)
3. Finish with arms locked and a 15- to 30-degree angle.
4. Return to starting position.

Reach failure between six and eight reps, no sandbagging. Rest two to three minutes between supersets.

**Hold the contracted extended position for one second; go as heavy as possible without sacrificing form.

*** Work up to a true three-repetition maximum. Rest two to three minutes between sets.

Day 5
Exercise Sets/Reps
Bodyweight Isometric Abductions *5/8

This is in the spirit of active recovery, but some serious muscle building will still take place.

*You will be in and out of the gym quickly today; rest 90 seconds between sets. Lift arms straight out to the side, fully extended. From this position contract the shoulders as hard as possible isometrically. Hold this position for six seconds, then relax. Repeat for a total of eight repetitions, and rest five seconds between repetitions.

Day 6
Repeat Day 1 with 80 percent intensity. All sets and reps are the same; use 80 percent of the weight you used Day 1. This is a stimulation workout. Rest two minutes between sets.

Day 7
Repeat Day 3

SHOCK TRAINING FOR BICEPS
There is a degree of truth to the clichéd expression: "Curls are for the girls." And Oso learned the veracity of that phrase once he started his male revue in and around Tijuana. Although Oso was not gifted with what most would call a "traditional male stripper build," he was almost childlike in his determined

desire to receive validation in the form of a drunken crowd of female bar patrons shouting his name with glee and desire in their voices.

To make his dream of emotional validation through male stripping a reality, Oso would implement any necessary change to his diet and training. One thing he found was that bigger and more defined biceps translated into more *pesos* in his briefs.

The workout described below is a variation of the shock training program for biceps that Oso used to become the "Most Improved Male Stripper" in Old Mexico.

Day 1
Exercise Sets/Reps
Cheat Curls 3/5*
One Arm Eccentric Barbell Curls**4/3
Gironda Perfect Curls***3/15, until failure, until failure

*This is not a wild heave; use just enough hip swing to get past the sticking point. From the fully contracted position, take five seconds to lower the weight to the starting position (arms fully extended). During the five-second negative, make a concerted effort to feel the bicep working. Go as heavy as possible without sacrificing technique or tempo. Rest two minutes between sets.

** Use full range of motion and go as heavy as possible. Using a full-length Olympic barbell, start from the bottom position with the arm you are working centered on the barbell. Have a partner or use your off arm to lift the weight to the fully contracted position. From this position, use the single arm you are working to lower the barbell to the starting position where the arms are extended (this will take eight seconds at a steady pace). Go as heavy as possible without sacrificing tempo. All of the work is on the eccentric, so get as much help as possible on the concentric. Rest one minute between arms and two minutes between sets.

***Start with your 15 rep max and perform for 15 reps. Rest one minute perform the same weight again to failure, rest one minute and do the same thing with the same weight. Subsequent sets will be performed for fewer reps. Maintain good form on all sets.

Day 2
Exercise Sets/Reps
Machine Curls 5/10*

This day is performed in the spirit of active recovery.

*Pick your favorite machine curl variation. Perform with half of the weight you would normally do for 10 reps. Do this for five sets and rest one minute between sets.

Day 3
Exercise Sets/Reps
Chin-up 5/5*

Incline Dumbbell Curls 5/10**
Hammer Curls 1/100***

The Chin-up and Incline Dumbbell Curl are examples of the concept of an origin/insertion superset. The origin is the fixed joint that doesn't move and the insertion is the joint that moves. Perform each exercise in succession with no rest. Rest three minutes between supersets.

*Chin-up means a supinated (underhand) grip. The biceps aids in this function. Go as heavy as possible with each set. If you can strap on extra weight, do it! Each set should be taken to the limit with a full range of motion.

**Make sure each rep is performed with a full range of motion. Fully contract at the top for half a second, and emphasize the stretch at the bottom. Go as heavy as possible without sacrificing technique.

***Use 25 percent of the weight you would normally use for a set of 10. Perform in a double armed action for 100 reps. If you reach failure before 100 reps, a slight cheat is okay. Excessive cheating is not allowed. If needed, rest for 20 seconds and continue. Repeat that sequence until 100 reps is reached.

Day 4
Exercise Sets/Reps
Isometric Biceps Curls *8/4

This is in the spirit of active recovery, but some serious muscle building will still take place.

*You will be in and out of the gym quickly today; rest 90 seconds between sets and five seconds between reps. Flex your biceps as hard as possible, forcing a maximal isometric contraction. Hold this for five seconds. Perform for four sets of eight repetitions.

Day 5
Repeat Day 2

Day 6
Exercise Sets/Reps
Gironda Perfect Curl 3/5*
Hammer Curls 3/6**

We are going as heavy as possible, but without any cheating whatsoever! Volume is low and the rest periods are long. The goal is to work up to a five rep max on the Gironda perfect curl and a six rep max on the hammer curl. Each set should be as close to the absolute maximum you can lift without technical break down.

*Rest three minutes between sets.

**Rest three minutes between sets

Day 7
Repeat Day 5

SHOCK TRAINING FOR TRICEPS

When you work the door of any bar, pub, or night club, there are times when you must get physical. Sometimes you are hauling a drug dealer out from the bathroom, other times you are tackling an enterprising patron who is running off with the liquor order, and there are instances when you are squaring off with a "trustee of modern chemistry" who is looking to try his luck with the doorman.

When Chaturo started working the door, he found that many times all that was necessary for the resolution of a conflict was a dynamic shove. If the timing and technique was right, he could push an unruly customer through the door and onto the street. Given the frequency with which he used this movement, Charuto trained his triceps, specifically so that he could propel the unwelcomed patron for the greatest distance possible.

The shock training program for triceps (described below) is taken from the method Charuto used to develop power for his barroom shove.

Day 1
Exercise Sets/Reps
Dips 3/5*
Close Grip Bench Press**2/5
Skull Crusher/Close Grip Bench Press 3/5***

*Stay upright to keep the emphasis on the triceps. On the first two sets, the weight should be one shy of failure. Select a weight with which you are able to complete six reps. On the final set, go to failure. Upon failure, we will continue with eccentrics. Boost yourself back to an arms locked position and lower yourself for a five second negative until your upper arms are parallel to the floor. Do this for four reps past failure. Rest two to three minutes between sets.

**Each set is a maximum weight to failure. Rest two to the three minutes between sets.

***Do a weight 10 percent above your heaviest skull crusher. Lower the weight as if performing a skull crusher for a five-second eccentric. Bring the weight from the bottom position to your chest press and close grip bench press the weight back to the starting point. Repeat this sequence five times. This is a hellacious eccentric overload. Rest two minutes between sets.

Day 2
Exercise Sets/Reps
Single-arm cable pushdowns* 5/15
The single arm (unilateral work) can help offset potential strength imbalances and the cable provides continuous tension on the movement while being very joint friendly.

*You will be in and out of the gym quickly today. Hold each rep in the bottom position for half a second, emphasizing the triceps contraction. Use a weight with which you are capable of doing 20 reps.

These should not be taken to failure. Rest one to two minutes between sets.

Day 3
Close-Grip Push-ups 5/50% of max *
Isometric Squeeze 5/15 Seconds **

You will be your own gym today! Because of the extreme methods used on Day 1, we will use only bodyweight and not approach failure.

*Rest 120 seconds between sets. Do 50 percent of the maximum reps you could do for one set. If you can do 30 push-ups, you will be doing sets of 15. Purposely emphasize triceps contraction on each rep. Use a grip with hands six inches apart. Rest two minutes between sets.

**Immediately after each set of close-grip push-ups, stand and extend your arms to the side of your body. Squeeze the triceps as hard as possible for 15 seconds.

Day 4
Exercise Sets/Reps
Dip 3/6-8 *
Overhead Rope Ext 3/12**
Kaz Press Smith Machine 3/6 ***

The dips and overhead rope extensions are a superset. Both exercises should be done as heavy as possible.

This is an origin/insertion superset—the origin is the fixed joint that doesn't move and the insertion is joint that moves—for dips the elbow is the origin, and for overhead rope triceps extension the shoulder is the origin. Supersetting an exercise for the same muscle with an origin, and insertion exercise is supersetting on an intense level. A muscle is attacked at different angles and by using different functions.

* and ** ***Rest two to three minutes between sets.

*Reach failure between six and eight reps, no sandbagging. Rest two to three minutes between supersets.

**Hold the contracted extended position for one second; go as heavy as possible without sacrificing form.

*** The Kaz Press is a hybrid close grip/triceps extension performed on a Smith machine. Rest two to three minutes between sets.

Day 5
Exercise Sets/Reps
Bodyweight Triceps Extensions * 5/10

This is a bodyweight movement in the spirit of active recovery.

*You will be in and out of the gym quickly today. Rest 90 seconds between sets. Position yourself at a spot where you are capable of doing 20 reps. Leverage is the key to intensity manipulation—the further your feet are away from the bar where you place your hands on, the more difficult the movement and the movement is easiest with feet on the floor. As feet are elevated, difficulty increases.

Day 6
Repeat Day 1 with 80 percent intensity. All sets and reps are the same, but use 80 percent of the weight you used on Day 1. If you weigh 160 pounds and performed dips with an extra 40 pounds added to your bodyweight (160+40=200), you will be using just your bodyweight this go around.

This is a stimulation workout. Rest two minutes between sets.

Day 7
Repeat Day 3

SHOCK TRAINING FOR FOREARMS
When Charuto worked the bars of Old Tijuana, he found that there were long periods where he could reflect. If there were no fights or none of his services was needed, Charuto filled those hours with a rich internal monologue. Part of that cerebral processing grew from observation. Like an anthropologist, Charuto would sit and observe the bar patrons.

One of the things he noticed was that the men who were the most physically dominant had a certain pattern to their body makeup. They had thick necks, wide upper backs, and muscular forearms. They had functional builds. If there was a fight later in the night, with rare exception, the functional man would be on the winning end.

In contrast to these men, there were the guys with fashionable builds (lightly toned arms and flat, but not necessarily muscular, tummies). These fashionable guys dressed in the latest styles and had girls who were similarly fashion-conscious. The girls were all smiles and giggles in the beginning of the night, but by the end of an evening some altercation or other barroom activity would inevitably leave them crying. Or worse yet, one would create drama for her date and the fashionable guy would fawn all over her attempting to resolve an irresolvable problem. If there was a barroom brawl, these fashionable guys would usually lose and their fancy clothes would be torn askew. Whether fighting with their dates or with another patron, the fashionable guys would often crack under pressure.

Charuto saw that the functional man also had dates. His dates were not made up with loud clothes or hiding behind flashy jewels, but they had a natural beauty. The functional man's date was smiles when she entered the bar and laughter when she left at the end of the evening. If there was a fight, she stood by her man (without tears). The functional man's clothing was different too. Where the fashionable guy's fancy dress attire would not withstand a barroom brawl, the functional man wore clothes that would bear hardship. From his clothes to his date to his body, the functional man is built to endure.

Charuto made a conscious decision to emulate many of the characteristics of the functional man. When he finally made some money and was able to buy new clothes, he shopped for quality clothing, like the functional man wore, and stayed away from the flashy items favored by the fashionable guy.

Charuto did not let too much get in the way of his training. But he would occasionally take a girl for a night out in Tijuana. When Charuto did date, he had no time for the girls easily distracted by flashy objects. Rather, he choose women who did not fall victim to their emotions and would appreciate the simple things in life like a fine single malt scotch, strong coffee, and the color of the morning sky after a long night with Charuto.

When Charuto made workouts, he placed a particular emphasis on functional muscles and movements. From this perspective, one of the most important muscles to develop are the forearms. Grabbing, throwing, grappling, lifting, and dragging all require forearm strength. To develop this crucial muscle group, Charuto would use a shock method program like the one below.

Day 1
Exercise Sets/Reps
Reverse Curls 5/5 *
Zottman Curls **

Since these exercises do not isolate the forearms, you have to go as heavy as possible.

* Maintaining good form, go as heavy as possible with a five-second negative on reverse curls. Rest two minutes between sets.

**Perform Zottman Curls by following these steps:

1. Stand up with your torso upright and a dumbbell in each hand held at arm's length. The elbows should be close to the torso.
2. Make sure the palms of the hands are facing each other. This will be your starting position.
3. While holding the upper arm stationary, curl the weights while contracting the biceps as you breathe out. Only the forearms should move. Your wrist should rotate so that you have a supinated (palms up) grip. Continue the movement until your biceps are fully contracted and the dumbbells are at shoulder level.
4. Hold the contracted position for a second as you squeeze the biceps.
5. Now during the contracted position, rotate your wrist until you have a pronated (palms facing down) grip with the thumb at a higher position than the pinky.
6. Slowly begin to bring the dumbbells back down using the pronated grip.

7. As the dumbbells come close your thighs, start rotating the wrist so that you go back to a neutral (palms facing your body) grip.
8. Repeat for the recommended amount of repetitions.

Go as heavy as possible and use "fat gripz," if available. Rest 90 seconds between sets.

Day 2
Exercise Sets/Reps
Dumbbell Wrist Curl 4/15*
Dumbbell Wrist Extension 4/15**

Keep form strict and emphasize a full range of motion. * and ** Both exercises should be done in a superset fashion. Rest one to two minutes between supersets.

Day 3
Exercise Sets/Reps
Newspaper Roll 5 sets

Due to the loading from the last couple of days, we are going to do an active recovery day and make it fun. Roll a newspaper as tight as possible in your hands for 30 seconds straight, rest 90 seconds and repeat. Emphasize squeezing the forearms.

Day 4
Exercise Sets/Reps
Towel Hangs 15 seconds, four sets

Time to build some grip strength. Size without strength is like a monster truck with a four-cylinder engine.

Throw a towel over a pull-up bar. Hang from the towel for 15 seconds. Rest two minutes between sets. This should be difficult. If it is easy, add weight to your body. If it is too difficult, partially support your weight by placing your feet on a bench or similar object.

Day 5
Exercise Sets/Reps
Ulna Deviation 5/15

Forearms do more than just extend and flex the wrist—they abduct (move away from body) and adduct (move toward the body). For complete development, we will work these functions.

*With the wrist, move the dumbbell toward the midline of the body by moving the little finger side of the hand toward the medial side of the forearm. Go as heavy as possible and use strict form because this is an isolation exercise. Rest one minute between sets.

Day 6
Exercise Sets/Reps
Radial Deviation 5/15

*This is a lateral movement away from the midline of the body done by moving the dumbbell from the thumb side of the hand toward the lateral side of the forearm. Go as heavy as possible and use strict form. Rest one minute between sets.

Day 7
Repeat Day 3

SHOCK TRAINING FOR CALVES

In the glory days of the Tijuana Barbell Club, lifting in Mexico was in its infancy. Not a lot of folks lifted and those who did focused on arms and chest. They wanted to look good for the *chicas* down at the beaches.

Kirk Peters was different. His pursuit of perfection led him to strive for the Grecian ideal, which is a concept of the human body established in Greek sculpture in the fifth century BCE. The Grecian ideal is characterized by clean and harmonious lines that join together in a well-proportioned body. When this is achieved, there remains an implicit and coiled movement inside of the body.

As Kirk's naturally broad shoulders became broader and his muscular arms popped the seams of his polo shirt, he became alert to lagging body parts. In particular, he noticed that his calves could be developed further and he turned to Charuto to construct a shock method program like the one below.

Day 1
Exercise Sets/Reps
Donkey Calf Raises 5/8 *

*Perform Donkey Calf Raises by following these steps:

1. For this exercise you will need access to a donkey calf raise machine. Start by positioning your lower back and hips under the padded lever provided. The tailbone area should make contact with the pad.

2. Place both of your arms on the side handles and place the balls of your feet on the calf block with the heels extending off. Align the toes forward, inward or outward, depending on the area you wish to target, and straighten the knees without locking them. This will be your starting position.

3. Raise your heels as you breathe out by extending your ankles as high as possible and flexing your calf. Ensure that the knee is kept stationary at all times. There should be no bending at any time. Hold the contracted position by a second before you start to go back down.

4. Go back slowly to the starting position as you breathe in, by lowering your heels as you bend the ankles until calves are stretched.

5. Repeat for the recommended amount of repetitions.

Pause two seconds at the top and two seconds at the bottom. Go as heavy as possible without sacrificing range of motion. Rest two minutes between sets.

Day 2

Exercise Sets/Reps

Seated Calf Raises 5/50, 40, 30, 20, 10 *

*Use a weight you can do 50 reps with on the first set. Rest two minutes between sets with a goal of using the same weight for all five sets without sacrificing technique.

Day 3

We will use the same exercise as Day 2 with the same sets and reps but with only 70 percent of the weight for Day 3. This is an active recovery day but with a good amount of volume and stimuli.

Day 4

Exercise Sets/Reps

Standing Calf raises (2 up, 1 down) 5/6*

One of the reason most folks' calf development is sub-par is because they do not train with eccentric emphasis movements. We don't care about traditions—we want results!

*Perform a standing full range of motion calf raise. From the top plantar flexed position, lower yourself to the bottom position, using only one leg with a steady five-second eccentric. Use as much weight as possible. A good starting point is a weight you can comfortably perform 15-20 reps with two legs in a traditional fashion. Rest two to three minutes between sets.

Day 5

Exercise Sets/Reps

Banded Tibia Raises 5/30*

Leaving no stone unturned, we will be performing band tibia raises, which work the tibialis anterior.

*Perform banded tibia raises by following these steps:

1. Loop a resistance band around a bench.
2. Stand at the edge and place one foot on the bench
3. Loop the band around the middle of your foot, making sure that there is tension in the band when stretched between your foot and the bench.
4. Flex your foot by pulling your toes toward you.
5. Pause, then return to the starting position. Repeat, then switch legs.
6. Repeat for desired number of reps.

Focus on keeping the movement strict at the ankle. Rest one to two minutes between sets.

Day 6

Exercise Sets/Reps

Calf Presses on Leg Press 5/15*

*Go as heavy as possible without sacrificing technique. Rest one to two minutes between sets.

Day 7
Exercise Sets/Reps
Single Leg Seated Dumbbell Calf Raises 5/30*

*Place a 2x4 board 12 inches in front of the bench you are sitting on. Rest one to two minutes between sets.

SHOCK TRAINING FOR QUADRICEPS
When Sugar Murray coerced Charuto into joining a strongman show, Charuto did not expect that the experience would morph into a travelling vaudevillian spectacle. Murray, the consummate hustler, thought that they could get a following if they travelled to Nogales, Juarez, and Monterrey.

For the most part, Charuto could read people well. It was a trait cultivated by his time working the door, where he would be required to make a quick judgement about someone's violent intentions. However, he would always believe in Murray's scatterbrained plans and it was no different when Murray suggested this itinerant idea.

To prepare for this next stage in the strongman show, Charuto need to develop his leg training beyond the rest pause routine. So he created the shock training workout for quadriceps, like the one included below.

Day 1
Exercise Sets/Reps
Front Squats 5/5*

Front squats are more knee-dominant than back squats. In other words, the quads are more active.

*Start light. The second set should increase in weight. The third set should be your top weight and maintain that weight for the remaining two sets. Rest three to four minutes between sets.

Day 2
Exercise Sets/Reps
Tyson Squat Workout* (see description)

Bodyweight squats force you to sit deeper, use your back less, and torch your quads in the process. Furthermore, reps with just your bodyweight will facilitate active recovery.

*Start with 10 playing cards and line them up two to four inches apart. Squat and pick up the first card, then move to the next card and place the first card on top of the second card. After which, you squat twice more to pick up each card individually, before moving to the third card. Walk to the third card and squat twice to stack each card, then squat three times to pick up each card before carrying the cards to the fourth card, and proceed with the pattern. You will continue this pattern of individually stacking and picking up the cards until you move through 10 ten cards in the line. At that point, you will have completed 100 squats. You can add cards as your strength and endurance increase.

Day 3

Exercise Sets/Reps

Toes Pointed in Leg Extensions 5/10

Squatting variations are functional and do a great job of inner quad or "tear drop" development, but they don't cut the mustard in developing "the sweep" or vastus lateralis.

No human movements isolate the quads from the hamstrings, but a large sweep is the ideal in body-building circles. So to acquire the sweep, you have to step outside of the functional training paradigm and hit the leg extensions. This unnatural movement unnaturally overloads the sweep to fully develop the quads and vastus lateralis.

To further accentuate the vastus lateralis, we will point the toes in while performing leg extensions. Per Tesch, MRI scans in the 1990s showed that pointing the toes in better isolate the vastus lateralis and more recent EMG studies confirm this.

*Use a tempo of three seconds on the eccentric, two seconds on the concentric, and hold at the top contracted position for one second. Go heavy but do not sacrifice technique or tempo for additional weight.

Day 4

Exercise Sets/Reps

Olympic Pause Squats 3/8 *

2 Up, 1 Down Leg Press 3/5**

Olympic lifters have some of the best tear drops in the business. Let's emulate their success and squat like an Olympic lifter. Pause at the bottom so the muscles are forced to do the work, rather than using the stretch shortening cycle to assist us out of the "hole." Furthermore, the pause will prolong time under tension. As we know, no muscle will fully develop without heavy eccentric work.

*Squat as low as possible. Think "ass to grass," not just breaking parallel. Pause each rep at the bottom for one second. Go as heavy as possible. Rest three to four minutes between sets.

**Use full range of motion. Start with a weight that you can do 20 reps with in a two-legged leg press. Lower with one leg for a steady tempo of five seconds. From the bottom position, forcefully push up to the starting position and repeat. Rest three minutes between sets.

Day 5
Repeat Day 2

Day 6
Exercise Sets/Reps
Sissy Squats 3/15 *
Toes Pointed in Leg Extensions 2/10**

*Get a good stretch at the bottom to reap the benefits of this movement. Use your bodyweight. Do not add additional resistance. Rest one to two minutes between sets.

**Use a tempo of three seconds on the eccentric, two seconds on the concentric, and hold at the top contracted position for one second. Go heavy, but do not sacrifice technique or tempo for additional weight. Rest 90 seconds between exercises.

Day 7
Exercise Sets/Reps
Pistol Squats 5/8 *

*If you are unable to complete pistol squats, do them on a bench or holding a squat rack. Once that becomes too easy, do them holding a towel. Rest one to two minutes between sets.

SHOCK TRAINING FOR HAMSTRINGS
Along with building his quadriceps for the myriad of bizarre strongman events devised by Sugar Murray, Charuto devised a shock training program for his hamstrings. This increased leg strength helped Charuto navigate his way through the odd shows of strength concocted by Murray in an attempt to attract as much attention as possible to their increasingly bizarre strength display.

When Chaurto's back legs became bigger and more defined, Murray suggested that Charuto perform the show in briefs to entice the female glance. According to Chato, there were still some old *senoras* who sigh when you remind them of the sight of Charuto in those briefs. There are also some old *senors* who remember the crazy strength show. The memories of both are driven by the increased hamstring strength developed from the shock method program similar to the one included below.

Day 1
Exercise Sets/Reps
Romanian Deadlift 3/5*
Lying 2 up, 1 down Leg Curl**3/4
Nordic Leg Curls Curl 3/3***

*Perform each rep as explosively as possible on the concentric. Envision a front to back movement, not an up and down one. Go as heavy as possible without sacrificing technique. Rest two to three minutes between sets.

** Use full range of motion and start with a weight that you can do 10 reps with in a two-legged leg lying leg curl. Lower with one leg for a steady tempo of five seconds. From the bottom position, forcefully curl to the starting position with two legs and repeat. Rest two minutes between sets and 45 seconds between legs.

***This is another eccentric emphasis movement. Perform these with a five-second eccentric, and then push yourself back to the starting position. If these are too difficult, use a resistance band for assistance.

Day 2
Exercise Sets/Reps
Good Mornings* 2/20
Seated Leg Curls **10/5

This day is primarily to facilitate the recovery process.

*Good Mornings are performed with 10-15 percent of your max squat. Emphasize the stretch. Rest one to two minutes between sets.

***Use half of the weight you would normally do for a set of 10. Rest one minute between sets.

Day 3
Repeat Day 2

Day 4
Exercise Sets/Reps
One Leg Romanian Dumbbell Deadlift *3/3
Romanian Deadlift**3/6
Lying Leg Curl***3/8

The Romanian Deadlift and lying leg curl are performed immediately after each other in a superset fashion. Rest three minutes between supersets. This is an origin/insertion superset (this is when the origin is the fixed joint that doesn't move and the insertion is joint that moves). With Romanian Deadlifts the knees are the origin, and for lying leg curls the hips are the origin.

*This is a favorite of former Canadian sprinter and world-record holder Ben Johnson, who performed this exercise with 110 pound dumbbells. Go as heavy as possible, while maintaining proper technique. Rest 90 seconds between sets and 45 seconds between legs.

**Go as heavy as possible while maintaining great form.

***Go as heavy as possible while maintaining great form.

Day 5
Exercise Sets/Reps
Isometric Leg Curls *6/4

This is in the spirit of active recovery but some serious muscle building will still take place.

*You will be in and out of the gym quickly today. Rest 90 seconds between sets. Lying on your stomach, flex your legs 15 degrees in this position and contract hamstrings as hard as possible. Hold this position for five second, relax, and repeat for a total of four repetitions. Rest eight seconds between repetitions and 90 seconds between sets. Repeat this at 60 and

90 degrees of leg flexion, following the exact same instructions.

Day 6
Exercise Sets/Reps
Glute Ham Raise *Undetermined/2

The glute ham raise is the ultimate hamstring builder. It forces an origin/insertion superset to take place with one movement! We will be in and out of the gym quickly today.

*Do two repetitions, emphasize perfect form, and explode through the concentric as hard as possible. Rest 20 seconds, repeat this process for six minutes, and perform quality reps. If these are very easy, you can put on a weighted vest or hold a plate. The workout is about six minutes in duration. Due to the low quantity, be sure to focus on the quality of the workout.

Day 7
Repeat Day 5

CONCLUSION

Every great story starts with an ending. The conclusion of our time learning under Chato was bittersweet. Our high school days were coming to an end and we were off to college, where we would be roommates and compete in athletics. While we were somewhat pensive about leaving our hometown, our gym, and our teacher, we were excited to start the next chapter in our lives.

On the day we were leaving for college, there was an unusual late summer marine layer hovering over our beach town. The fog seemed to reflect our mood as we stepped into the gym for one last workout. Unsurprisingly, Chato was there, putting in some time with the iron.

As soon as Chato saw us, he walked over with the cool, confident gait of one who carried the last remnants of that inspirational spark that created the lost bodybuilding era of Old Mexico.

"So, today is the big day? Off to college and the big world?"

"Yep."

"Are you guys excited?"

"Yes," we replied with a slight shoulder shrug.

"Oh. Then, why the long faces?"

"Well, I guess we are a little sorry to leave the gym and we will miss hearing your stories."

Chato paused and it seemed that he was not used to the emotion that his usually stoic face revealed.

He almost seemed strained when he responded. "You guys have done me a tremendous service. You listened and learned. There are few greater ways for a younger generation to honor those who came before. Now, I ask a favor of you. One day, when you guys have an audience, and I know that you will have an audience, share the story of the Tijuana Barbell Club."

"We can do that."

"I know you can and you will. Listen, don't be anxious about this time in your life coming to a conclusion. *Every great story starts with an ending.* By finishing this period in your life, it is now time to write the next chapter in your story."

With those words we turned the page from that time in our lives, but we always remembered Chato, Charuto, Kirk Peters, Oso, and the Saga of the Tijuana Barbell. It has served us a source of inspiration, entertainment, and improvement. May it do the same for you.

Made in United States
Troutdale, OR
01/26/2024

17172130R00076